THE
HEALING
HERBS
COOKBOOK

PAT CROCKER

FOREWORD BY JAMES A. DUKE
AUTHOR OF *THE GREEN PHARMACY*

Robert
ROSE

THE HEALING HERBS COOKBOOK

DESIGN, EDITORIAL AND PRODUCTION:	MATTHEWS COMMUNICATIONS DESIGN INC.
PHOTOGRAPHY:	MARK T. SHAPIRO
ART DIRECTION/FOOD PHOTOGRAPHY:	SHARON MATTHEWS
FOOD STYLIST:	KATE BUSH
PROP STYLIST:	CHARLENE ERRICSON
RECIPE EDITORS/TEST KITCHEN:	RIKI DIXON/JAN MAIN
MANAGING EDITOR:	PETER MATTHEWS
INDEXER:	BARBARA SCHON
COLOR SCANS & FILM:	POINTONE GRAPHICS

We acknowledge the financial support of the Government of Canada through the Book Publishing Industry Development Program (BPIDP) for our publishing activities.

Canadä

Canadian Cataloguing in Publication Data

Crocker, Pat L.

The healing herbs cookbook

Includes index.
ISBN 0-7788-0004-0

1. Cookery (Herbs). 2. Herbs – Therapeutic use. I. Title.

TX819.H4C76 1999   641.6'57   C99-930016-4

Published by: Robert Rose Inc. • 156 Duncan Mill Road, Suite 12
Toronto, Ontario, Canada M3B 2N2 Tel: (416) 449-3535

Printed in Canada

1234567 BP 02 01 00 99

Contents

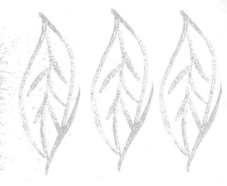

ACKNOWLEDGEMENTS

After more than a decade of country living, growing, learning, writing and teaching about herbs, I have come to see these simple plants as a symbol of hope for mankind. It is to all these humble plants — which offer their great resources in order that we may live with continuing good health and well-being — that I owe the greatest debt.

My love of food and my cooking style has evolved thanks to some special people. Not long after we moved to the rich land around the Saugeen River, Ruth and Doug MacDonald shared their love of family, friends and food with us. Doug introduced me to wild leeks, while Ruth's gentle way with plants and gardens inspired me to keep working at my own, meager garden skills. Their "smoky" maple syrup is still the best I've ever tasted.

Many of the recipes in this book were developed and tested with biodynamically grown vegetables provided by the hard work of Holly MacKay and Corey Eichman, who run the Saugeen River Community Supported Agriculture program near Durham, Ontario. Here are two young people working at what they love with a sense of pride and social consciousness. Bravo to them and all the other dedicated organic stewards of one of the earth's most precious resources.

Thanks also to Conrad Richter for his support and help in offering the use of his extensive herb library. Susan Eagles has been a tremendous support for the technical information on medicinal herbs. Her help is greatly appreciated.

Pat Crocker

PHOTO PROP CREDIT

The publisher and authors wish to express their appreciation to the following supplier of props used in the food photography appearing in this book:

Dishes, cutlery, glassware, linens and accessories: **URBAN MODE**

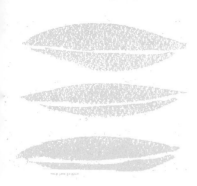

Foreword by James A. Duke

Many decades of pleasurable lab and field research with medicinal plants — on many continents, with both primitive and modern peoples — have convinced me that numerous herbal medicines are safer and cheaper than (if not as efficacious as) the pharmaceuticals promoted so vigorously here in North America. These plants — some appearing in our foods, especially as herbs and spices — are often loaded with biologically active compounds with which our genes evolved over the millennia. Our genes, like our bodies, not only recognize many of the phytochemicals in these empirically selected culinary plants, they may actually need some of them.

Only in 1998 did we realize that choline, found in most of our plants, is essential to health — so much so that we established a recommended daily allowance (RDA) for it. More such discoveries will be made as we approach the new millennium.

There are many compounds that our ancestors ingested in greater quantity (and sometimes variety) than we do today. Yet the United States Department of Agriculture (USDA) is busily breeding out such compounds. In the case of soybeans, for example, there are at least five cancer-preventive "antinutrients" that are being removed by plant breeders. Food-processing companies remove even more compounds — often the same necessary phytochemicals that they will be selling us as nutritional supplements tomorrow.

During my decades with the USDA as a botanist and ecologist (from which I evolved into an ethnobotanist), I developed an extensive database of published scientific information about the various chemicals and compounds found in food and medicinal plants. It is pleasing to see that in The Healing Herbs Cookbook, Pat Crocker has drawn upon the growing body of scientific research surrounding those chemicals as they relate to the health of human beings.

In profiling over 30 healing herbs, she has demystified those herbs for cooks, gardeners, health practitioners and all kinds of people from all walks of life who want their food to reflect a healthy lifestyle. The combination of fresh air, exercise and a well-balanced, phytochemical-laden diet is essential to health, and actually prevents many of the chronic diseases that synthetic pharmaceuticals try to correct. Lifestyle — including a balanced diet of whole foods, exercise, hard work, meditation and contemplation — is the first defense. Obey your body and you won't have to resort to so many of the questionable offerings promoted by pharmaceutical companies.

With her focus on healthy eating, Pat Crocker's message (and I agree with it) is that humans will function optimally and with a reduced risk of the diseases that plague modern society if they build their diet around whole, live, organic grains, legumes, fruits, vegetables, nuts, seeds and herbs. She presents her information in a clear, concise format with a view to the practical aspects of buying, preparing, cooking with and enjoying herbs.

There are many excellent "herbals" and even more top-notch cookbooks available today. Most good herb books offer well-researched information on herbs and herbal remedies. Some offer recipes and practical methods for using the healing herbs as medicinal therapies, while others — like my own book, **The Green Pharmacy** — are more comprehensive in their approach to applying herbs to specific health conditions. However, I would venture to say that no herbal and few cookbooks make the connection between healing herbs, specific health issues and recipes for everyday meals as directly and with as much downright good taste as **The Healing Herbs Cookbook**. More importantly, this book sets us on a new culinary course reminiscent of ancient Chinese and first American peoples' cooking traditions, passed down orally through the centuries. In short, it gets us back to thinking about medicinal herbs as food.

I enjoy eating, especially a wide variety of whole foods prepared fresh and first for me. When the foods that I eat have been combined with herbs that I know will benefit my body, I am truly in sync with the natural world with which we co-evolved.

When people ask me for recipes for food "farmaceuticals" and wholesome, delicious recipes, I'm usually nonplussed. Those of my recipes that you see giving measures have been coerced out of me by strident editors demanding a precision I lack. I never measure out a recipe — for a tea, for a soup, for a liqueur, for a stew, for a fruit or veggie smoothie — and yet I eat one or more of these items almost every day when I'm at home, trying to get (and usually getting) that "five and five" for which we strive to stay alive. But now, I'll be pleased to suggest Pat Crocker's informative and useful book, **The Healing Herbs Cookbook**.

Delightful!

James A. Duke
Economic Botanist (USDA, ret.)

Author of the USDA's phytochemical database
http://www.ars-grin.gov/duke/

and THE GREEN PHARMACY (Rodale Press)

INTRODUCTION

Better is a dinner of herbs where love is...
Proverbs

Remembering my parents, Bill and Vera Crocker.

Cod fish and brewis with scruntions for him and the pope's nose for her.

Thanks to them, it's a flavorful legacy I've inherited.

Cooking involves our bodies, minds and souls. Or at least, it does when we cook for the right reasons — whatever they might be for each of us. I cook because it is one of the ways to express my creative inventiveness and to make a personal gift to those I care about. I enjoy cooking because it is often a meditative time, a time when I am alone, when I can sort through a problem or think of new ideas for current projects.

For me, a table covered with wholesome food, surrounded by faces I love, is one of the threads that weaves magic into the fabric of our lives. It connects us to the land, to each other and to our spiritual heritage. Stopping to eat and talk and listen, to enjoy one another's company nourishes family and community life.

It's not a stretch to go from cooking for pleasure to cooking for health. At least, it wasn't for me. I planted my first herb garden because I wanted my recipes to reflect the vibrant taste that only fresh culinary herbs can give. From tarragon, thyme, sage, marjoram and the rest, I went to hyssop, calendula and ginseng, hardly skipping a beat. At first, I used medicinal herbs in traditional ways, making tinctures, salves, poultices, teas, syrups and oils. I was pleased with the way my herbal "simples" eased our life and I began to share what I had learned about healing herbs with others in my workshops, walks and lectures. I can't imagine a winter without Lavender-Calendula hand salve or St. John's Wort oil, but it wasn't long before I wondered why we couldn't use healing herbs in everyday meals. After all, some of the most medicinally potent herbs and spices sit within arm's reach — on the kitchen spice rack.

Not a lot has been written or studied about cooking with medicinal herbs. We don't know if heating for long periods of time damages some of the active ingredients in some herbs. In others, we don't even know the exact amount of vitamins and minerals they contain. So why bother to include them in our daily diet?

The answer lies in the basic concept that we eat to nourish our cells and ourselves. These days, that idea is sometimes forgotten in the whirlwind of busy lives, convenience foods and pick-up meals. Cooking with medicinal herbs supports the idea that we are responsible for our own health. By taking an interest in the way our food is grown and processed and in the way it is handled and prepared, served and enjoyed, we are participating in our nourishment and health. By choosing to cook with whole, fresh, organic ingredients as well as healing herbs, we are reinforcing with action a desire to be healthy. And that, alone, is a powerful act.

The intent of this book is to pique your interest in herbs, both culinary and medicinal. It is meant to provoke reflective thought about the connection between your health and the food choices you make. The recipes are offered in a spirit of healthy, life-sustaining, disease prevention. They are a wise alternative to today's over-refined, additive-laden fast foods. I do not recommend that you rely exclusively on these recipes if you are ill. Diagnosis and therapeutic use of medicinal herbs is best guided by a professional.

The recipes in this book are designed to give you many ways to present whole, "living" food in everyday meals. They follow, more or less, a macrobiotic diet for North Americans. That is, they use whole food which still contains its vitality and is seasonal and indigenous to our environment. Whole grains, vegetables and fruit (except those tropical), legumes and beans, small amounts of fish or organic meat, sea vegetables and nuts and seeds are foods that are appropriate for where we live.

As we reduce the meat and fat and fill up our plates with whole grains, legumes and vegetables, we will come to rely more and more on herbs. Fat as an ingredient is full of flavor and what food professionals call "mouthfeel." Cutting the fat in recipes can result in a bland imitation of the foods most people love. The food industry has met this challenge with a variety of artificial flavors, gums and other non-food additives. Home cooks, on the other hand, have a natural, life-supporting ingredient to fill the flavor gap — namely, fresh herbs.

The other happy result of using less refined foods is that dietary fiber — that delicious snap, crunch and chewy texture that comes only from fresh fruits and vegetables, unrefined grains and legumes — will reappear in our daily meals to help absorb toxins, keep us eliminating regularly and, most importantly, help to protect us from colon cancer.

You will not find bottled shortcuts, processed foods nor food in bags or boxes used in these recipes because there simply is no shortcut to good health. At the same time, I hope I have dished up ample servings of sensory pleasure because, in the end, cooking and eating should be joyful activities.

Eating fresh, dynamic, organic food is, I know, a personal challenge for each of us. However, the extent to which we meet that challenge will determine how vibrant and healthy we are. I encourage you to let your fork lead you to good health.

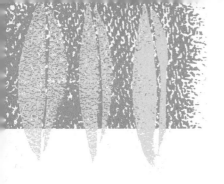

HERBS: THE HELPING PLANTS

If they would drink nettles in March
And eat mugwort in May,
So many fine maidens
Wouldn't go to the clay.
— Old Proverb

Herbs embody a simple life. Their roots intertwine with our culinary, mythical, cultural and medicinal heritage. Indeed, there once was a time when "garden" meant "herb garden," when both the vegetable and the flower garden were non-existent. Today, people are turning to herbs once again, for many reasons, not the least of which is their ability to reconnect us to nature.

HERBS AND HUMANITY

When we pull our hand along the piney stem of a rosemary bush, we pull the tenacious thread of our history, right back to the very dawn of man's emergence as a cultivator. Because, unlike contemporary crops and ornamentals, most herbs (including the rosemary plant of today) are the very same plants upon which kings, monks and ordinary folk would have performed that same fragrant ritual.

Indeed, they are the same plants that foraging early humans might have rubbed on their bodies — and, later, on their meat — to repel insects and preserve their food. In time, humans began adding roots, bark, leaves and flowers to stews, and using aromatic herbs to prevent illness or assist with healing. The next step was to control the growth of these important plants.

Herbs have been cultivated for 10,000 years, being the first of the plants to come under man's domination. Many herbs and spices figure prominently in ancient religions, including early Christianity. If we study the value people have placed on individual herbs throughout that time, we are offered a rare glimpse into the psyche of humans. Witness basil, which was revered and used in love spells by Iron-Age Celts, yet the ancient Greeks believed that it represented hate and misfortune and, later, people went so far as to say that basil bred scorpions, which formed in the brain if used as snuff.

If we look at how herbs were used, we unravel details about day-to-day life throughout our history. For example, right up until World War I, people scurried out in the spring to gather wild burdock, dandelion, and nettles to make tonics for cleansing the system. This practice evolved from centuries before, when fresh vegetables were virtually unknown during winter. The Lenten fast, followed by a dose of bitter Spring Tonic served to cleanse the body of all vestiges of tainted meat and helped to prepare it for the "shock" of fresh, raw produce.

The Lure of Herbs Today

The Herb Society of America defines herbs as "any plant that may be used for pleasure, fragrance or physic," and it is their role as life-enhancers that gives them such a broad appeal to people today. For the first half of the 20th century, science, technology and the rise of our urban culture caused a decline in popular interest and use of herbs. But with the new millennium upon us, those same developments are driving us to embrace these organic, earthy plants.

Herbs exist in our minds as well as in our gardens. Our balcony or backyard herb garden, no matter how small or simple, is our link to the great walled sanctuaries of long ago. In the herb garden, problems seem easier to solve, life is gentler and a sense of balance can be maintained. In the herb garden, Mother Earth takes center stage and the ancient right of man to use these plants for his own well-being comes to full fruition.

Herbs and a Holistic Lifestyle

Herbs are beginning to sprout back into modern culture. People with a concern about toxic chemicals in food are buying fresh, nutrient-rich organic herbs along with their fruits and vegetables, and so the vitamins, minerals and trace elements in herbs are once again contributing significantly to our diet. Cosmetics are now available that are not based on petrochemicals, but have as their base pure essential oils derived from herb flowers and leaves. The growing scientific evidence for the medicinal value of herbs is putting herbal remedies into mainstream consciousness. We often see recipes for gentle, homemade household cleaning products that rely on herbs and natural ingredients. Heck, we can even repel bugs by strictly herbal methods.

It's not long after the practical aspects of herbs are appreciated that their deeper meanings begin to affect our lives. The person who makes gifts of handmade pot pourri from herbs, flowers, spices and essential oils also benefits from the gift of time — precious meditative time spent collecting, preparing and handling these wonderful plants. Herbs allow us to draw on ancient rituals that once served to give people spiritual definition. Not surprising then that the Navajo smudge pot is finding widespread use among non-natives now. By learning about even just one herb's medicinal value and using it correctly, we make huge strides towards taking responsibility for our own health. Thus, what may have begun as simply a love of plants or a desire to grow some culinary herbs indoors, could very well result in a shift in the way we think about ourselves, our life and the world around us.

Herb Profiles

Alfalfa
Medicago sativa

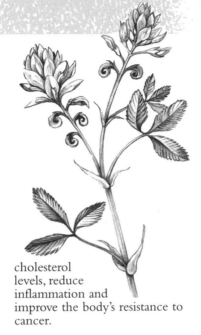

DESCRIPTION

An upright, extensively branched stem (1 to 3 feet [30 to 60 cm]) growing from a deep taproot which penetrates to a depth of up to 100 feet (30 m); has oval leaves, grouped in three. Blue or violet spike flowers appear from June to August.

FLAVOR

A light, "green" taste to the fresh flowers and leaves. A stronger, "grassy" taste to the dried aerial parts.

PARTS USED

Leaves, flowers and sprouted seeds.

HOW TO GROW

Type: hardy perennial
Exposure: full sun; average soil
Propagation: from seed or nursery plants
Harvest: aerial parts when in full flower, save and use seeds for planting and sprouting

HEALING PROPERTIES

Actions: tonic, nutritive, anti-cholesterol, anti-anemia

Uses: Alfalfa is a cell nutritive and overall tonic for the body, helping to maintain or regain health by feeding the cells; useful to build up the body in debility (such as after illness or surgery) and in arthritis. Nutrients in alfalfa promote strong teeth, bones and other connective tissue. Alfalfa is one of the best sources of chlorophyll, which has the ability to stimulate new skin growth, heal wounds and burns, diminish the symptoms of arthritis, gout and rheumatism, lower cholesterol levels, reduce inflammation and improve the body's resistance to cancer.

Phytochemistry: The mature tops and seeds are high in pantothenic acid, amino acids and chlorophyll, as well as minerals such as calcium, magnesium, phosphorus and potassium and vitamins K, B and P, which the body uses to repair and build musculoskeletal system structures and tissues. Sprouted seeds have an enhanced concentration of vitamins.
Food value (shoots, per 100 g): 3,410 I.U. beta carotene; 162 mg Vitamin C.

AVAILABILITY

Whole or cut, dried leaf available in alternative/health stores. Sprouted seeds readily available.

HOW TO USE IN COOKING

As a response to anticipated food shortages, alfalfa protein was originally developed as an emergency food for England during World War II. Not actually used then, it is now being introduced to communities in Mexico, Bangladesh, Bolivia, Sri Lanka, India, Ghana and Nicaragua.
Whole sprigs: fresh or dried, add to soups and stews during the last hour of cooking, then remove.
Leaf: fresh, in salads, rice and vegetable dishes. Use a generous handful of fresh or dried alfalfa in vegetable (or meat) stocks. Add chopped leaf to soups and stews during the last 10 minutes of cooking.
Flowers and Sprouts: fresh in salads, stir-fries and sandwiches; add when juicing vegetables; include with liquids in breads.
Use fresh or dried flowers and leaves blended with green tea for a nutritious daily drink.

FOLKLORE

Humanity's oldest crop, to the ancient Arabs, alfalfa was the "father of all foods" (al-fal-fa) and they used it as a nutritive staple. Alfalfa was introduced to California by gold prospectors in the 1850s, and was planted on the Minnesota plains by a German immigrant in 1857.

Astragalus
Astragalus membranaceus
(Huang Qi)

DESCRIPTION

A. membranaceus is one of about 2,000 species in the genus Astragalus, some of which are poisonous. Also called milk vetch, it is a shrub-like plant (to about 2 feet [60 cm]), with

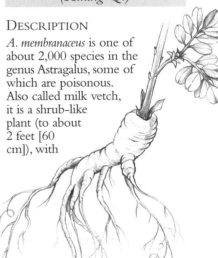

sprawling, hairy stems and alternate leaves divided into 12 to 20 elongated oval leaflets. Small yellow pea flowers produce 6-inch (15 cm) kidney-shaped pods in late summer. Long, woody slices of dried root are a light cream color.

FLAVOR
Mild, slightly sweet, earthy taste.

PARTS USED
Root.

HOW TO GROW
Type: a perennial native to eastern Asia but grown in temperate regions
Exposure: dry, sandy soil, full sun
Propagation: from seed in spring or fall
Harvest: roots are harvested in autumn, sliced and dried

HEALING PROPERTIES
Actions: Immunostimulant, antimicrobial, cardiotonic, diuretic, promotes tissue regeneration

Uses: Chinese astragalus root is widely used throughout the Orient as a tonic, food, and medicinal plant. It is a powerful immune system stimulator for virtually every phase of immune system activity. Research has documented that *A. membranaceus* increases the number of "stem cells" in the marrow and lymph tissue, and stimulates their development into active immune cells which are released into the body. Astragalus can promote or trigger immune cells from the "resting" state into heightened activity. It also has been shown to alleviate the adverse effects of steroids and chemotherapy on the immune system and stimulates the production of interferon and increases its effects in fighting disease.
Often used in combination with other Chinese herbs for the treatment of fatigue, heart disease and other ailments.

AVAILABILITY
Dried root, 6 to 12 inches (15 to 30 cm) long, available in Oriental markets, alternative/health stores.

HOW TO USE IN COOKING
Add to soups or soup stocks; grind and include in root beverages and seasoning blends.

FOLKLORE
The name Astragalus is derived from the ancient Greek meaning "ankle bone." Ankle bones were once used as dice and it is thought that the rattling of the seed pods of Astragalus was similar to the sound made by rolling the bones. Chinese use of *huang-qi* dates beyond 2,000 years.

Burdock
Arctium lappa

DESCRIPTION
Root is thick, brownish-grey on the exterior with white pith-like tissue inside. A dull-green hairy stem grows to 3 feet (90 cm) with large leaves. Small, red or purple flowers, resembling thistles, are set in distinctive fruiting heads covered with hooked burrs, appearing from late summer through the fall.

FLAVOR
Cooked root is sweet, similar to potato in flavor. Teas made from dried root have a pleasant, earthy, nutty flavor.

PARTS USED
Root, stalk & leaves, seeds.

HOW TO GROW
Type: hardy biennial
Exposure: full sun; light soil
Propagation: from seeds in burrs
Harvest: clip tender leaves in spring; dig roots in fall, after the first frost

HEALING PROPERTIES
Actions:
Root: mild laxative, antirheumatic, antibiotic, diaphoretic, diuretic, alterative, a skin and blood cleanser, burdock stimulates urine flow and sweating. Root and seeds are a soothing demulcent, tonic, soothe kidneys and relieve lymphatics.
Leaves: mild laxative, diuretic
Seeds: prevent fever, anti-inflammatory, antibacterial, reduce blood sugar levels

Uses: Burdock root is used as a cleansing, eliminative remedy. It helps to remove toxins causing skin problems (including eczema, acne, rashes, boils), digestive sluggishness, or arthritic pains. Leaves may be used for similar problems although less effective than the root.

Food value (boiled root, per 1 cup [250 mL]): 61 mg calcium; 450 mg potassium; 116 mg phosphorus

AVAILABILITY
This is an easy plant for North Americans to forage because of its widespread availability in rural and urban areas. (Avoid collecting from roadsides, ditches or streams close to field run-off and other areas of pollution.) Cut, dried root available in alternative/health stores.

HOW TO USE IN COOKING
Mrs. Grieve, in *A Modern Herbal*, tells us how to use burdock stalks, "...the stalks, cut before the flower is open and stripped of their rind, form a delicate vegetable when boiled, similar in flavor to Asparagus, and also make a pleasant salad, eaten raw with oil and vinegar. Formerly they were sometimes candied with sugar, as Angelica is now. They are slightly laxative, but perfectly wholesome"[2]

[2.] *A Modern Herbal*, Vol. I, by Mrs. M. Grieve, Dover Publications Inc., N.Y. 1971, p. 144

Leaves: wrap vegetables, fish and meat in fresh leaves for grilling. Use tender young sprouts and spring leaves in salads and soups or cooked as a vegetable.
Seeds: dry and include in tea blends.
Roots: use fresh roots and stalks in soups instead of potatoes; roast or grill roots as a vegetable, grate and mix with potatoes for latkes; roasted, dried roots as a coffee substitute.

FOLKLORE

Burdock was an important medicine for Native American tribes, particularly the Cherokee and Chippewa. It is from the Indians that Canadian Eileen Caisse learned their anti-cancer formula (which she called Essiac®) of which burdock is one of four herbal ingredients.

Calendula
Calendula officinalis

DESCRIPTION

A short (up to 18 inches [45 cm]), erect plant with strong, branching stems. Bright yellow, variegated and deep orange flowers (2 to 3 inches [5 to 7.5 cm] in diameter) in solitary, terminal heads.

FLAVOR

A delicate floral taste and smell. Flavor and aroma strengthens upon drying but is still overpowered by other robust ingredients in food.

PARTS USED

Petals.

HOW TO GROW

Type: hardy annual
Exposure: full sun; average soil
Propagation: from fresh seed; or transplant in spring, 18 inches (45 cm) apart; seed will self-sow
Harvest: early-mid summer when flowers are at their peak

HEALING PROPERTIES

Actions: astringent, antiseptic, anti-fungal, anti-inflammatory, heals wounds, menstrual regulator, stimulates bile production

Uses: Calendula acts as an aid to digestion and as a general tonic which makes it a good addition to all dishes. It is taken to ease menopausal problems, period pain, and gastritis.

AVAILABILITY

Whole dried flowerheads available in alternative/health stores.

HOW TO USE IN COOKING

Stevens, in *Maison Rustique*, or *the Countrie Farme* (1699) writes of calendula, "Conserve made of the flowers and sugar, taken in the morning fasting, cureth the trembling of the harte, and is also given in the time of plague or pestilence. The yellow leaves of the flowers [petals] are dried and kept throughout Dutchland against winter to put into broths, physicall potions and for divers other purposes, in such quantity that in some Grocers or Spicesellers are to be found barrels filled with them and retailed by the penny or less, insomuch that no broths are well made with out dried Marigold."[3] Formerly used to color cheese, calendula adds a soft, flecked yellow color to baked products, rice and sauces. Use it as a substitute for saffron and a natural food coloring. Use fresh petals chopped in salads, soups, stews, rice, egg dishes, custards and puddings; fresh or dried petals as a garnish for all main or dessert dishes, in cakes, breads and muffins, in non-alcoholic punches, in frozen ices and flower seasonings.

---

[3]. *Ibid*, Vol. II, p. 517

FOLKLORE

Calendula has a long history of culinary use from medieval times to the 18th century. Ancient Romans named this plant calendula because it bloomed on the first day, or *calends*, of every month. Legend claims that the Romans took marigold from India, where it originated, because they found it too difficult to carry saffron. In 1577, Thomas Hyll wrote that the juice of the petals with vinegar was to be rubbed on the gums and teeth and thought it "a soveraigne remedy for the assuaging of the grevious pain of the teethe."

Cayenne
Capsicum annum and *Capsicum frutescens*

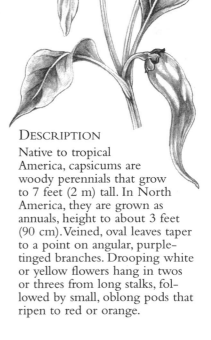

DESCRIPTION

Native to tropical America, capsicums are woody perennials that grow to 7 feet (2 m) tall. In North America, they are grown as annuals, height to about 3 feet (90 cm). Veined, oval leaves taper to a point on angular, purple-tinged branches. Drooping white or yellow flowers hang in twos or threes from long stalks, followed by small, oblong pods that ripen to red or orange.

FLAVOR
Hot, biting.

PARTS USED
Red pepper fruit.

HOW TO GROW
Type: annual (in North America)
Exposure: full sun; average soil
Propagation: plant seedlings in spring
Harvest: mid-late summer when fruit is ripe

HEALING PROPERTIES
Actions: stimulant, tonic, carminative, diaphoretic, rubefacient, antiseptic, anti-bacterial

Uses: Cayenne purifies the blood and promotes fluid elimination and sweat and is most often used as a stimulating nerve tonic. Applied externally, over-the-counter creams and ointments containing the active capsaicin extract are often effective in relieving the pain of osteoarthritis and rheumatoid arthritis, shingles infection, as well as the burning pain in the toes, feet, and legs of diabetic neuropathy and fibromyalgia (a painful musculoskeletal condition). Capsaicin is the most efficacious herbal derivative now used in the symptomatic treatment of arthritis.

Phytochemistry: Capsaicin works by blocking a protein called "substance P," which normally relays pain messages from nerve endings to the brain.

Food value (per 1 tbsp [15 mL]): 7.8 mg calcium; 0.4 mg iron, 8 mg magnesium, 15.5 mg phosphorus, 107 mg potassium, 4 mg vitamin C; 2,205 I.U. vitamin A.

CAUTION
Cayenne has an irritating property that, applied externally, heals unbroken inflammations by bringing the blood (with its nutrients) to the surface blood vessels. Its antiseptic properties are useful as a wash to clean open sores, and as a gargle for sore throat, but the healing process in broken skin will be inhibited by repeated application. Capsicum should not be used internally in cases of chronic inflammation of the intestinal tract, such as in Irritable Bowel Syndrome, Ulcerative Colitis and Crohn's Disease.

AVAILABILITY
Fresh, whole chili peppers available in some ethnic markets, supermarkets and alternative/health stores. Dried whole chilies, and powdered cayenne pepper are widely available.

HOW TO USE IN COOKING
Start with small doses — experts say that virtually everybody can gradually build up a tolerance to the hot taste and learn to love it. Milk, yogurt and ice cream soothe the tongue. Cayenne pepper is the principal ingredient of hot tabasco sauce.
Whole: fresh chilies, chopped, in tomato sauces, soups, stews, preserved in "chili" sauces; chopped, in raw or cooked salsas; roasted, peeled, chopped in sauces; dried, whole chilies in soups, soup stocks, crushed as a garnish for salads, cooked dishes, blended in teas.
Dried powdered: as a garnish for main dish meals and in spice blends and rubs for roasted or grilled meats and vegetables.

FOLKLORE
By the mid-16th century, Europeans were using capsicum as a local stimulant, gargle, and counterirritant liniment. Around 1790, Samuel Thomson used cayenne to "produce a strong heat in the body and to restore digestive powers. There is scarce any preparation of medicine that I make use of in which I do not put some of this article."
— self-styled physician Samuel Thomson (1769 - 1843).

Chamomile
Matricaria recutita (German) or *Chamaemelum nobile* (Roman)

DESCRIPTION
The Roman plant is low-growing but the German variety can grow to 2 1/2 feet (75 cm). A creeping hardy plant with mat-like stems and lacy, fern-like foliage, flowers are like small delicate white daisies with rounded yellow centers.

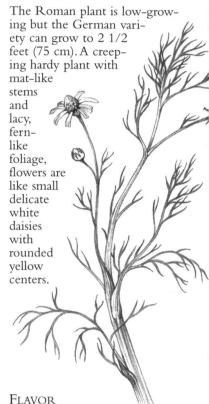

FLAVOR
Fragrant, apple-like taste.

PARTS USED
Flowerheads and petals.

HOW TO GROW
Type: hardy annual (the Roman variety is a perennial)
Exposure: full sun; moist, rich soil
Propagation: seeds or seedlings; self-sows easily
Harvesting: blooms develop continuously, and once flowering commences, harvest every 10 days to 2 weeks.

HEALING PROPERTIES
While German and Roman chamomile plants have been used interchangeably for medicinal or commercial purposes, the chemical composition of the flowers

and their essential oils is different. Healing properties and phytochemistry here are related to the German variety.

Actions: sedative, anti-inflammatory, anti-bacterial, prevents vomiting, antispasmodic, tonic stimulant, carminative, diaphoretic, nervine, emmenagogue

Uses: Anxiety, insomnia, indigestion, and inflammations (such as gastritis) are often eased with chamomile. Chamomile also reduces flatulence and pain caused by gas. Several chemical compounds in the essential oil of the plant have proved capable of relaxing smooth muscle tissue which supports its use as a spasm-relieving agent, primarily for menstrual cramps. German commercial products are used to alleviate minor pain, clean wounds, kill bacteria and treat skin or mouth infections.

Phytochemistry: To date, more than 120 chemical components have been identified from chamomile's clear blue essential oil. Chamazulene, alpha-bisabolol and matricinare are considered responsible for the primary medicinal activity of the herb — all three have been evaluated individually and found to reduce inflammation. Alpha-bisabolol is also strongly antispasmodic, antimicrobial and mildly sedative.

Food value (tea, brewed, 1 cup [250 mL]): 21 mg potassium, 47 I.U. vitamin A

CAUTION
Those allergic to pollen of members of the aster family (such as ragweed), may also be allergic to chamomile. According to Dr. Tyler, 50 allergic reactions were reported from 1887 to 1982; of these, only 5 were attributed to German chamomile.

AVAILABILITY
Whole dried flowerheads available in alternative/health stores.

HOW TO USE IN COOKING
Use chamomile to flavor jams, jellies, syrups and sauces. Fresh or dried petals may be used in salads and as edible garnish, in baked goods and other desserts such as puddings.
To relieve an acute upset stomach, take chamomile tea between meals on an empty stomach so the tea will have direct contact with the mucous lining.

FOLKLORE
The Greeks named the plant "ground apple" — *kamai* (on the ground) and *melos* (apple) — because of its low-growing characteristic and distinct apple fragrance. Known as the "ginseng of Europe," chamomile comprises 18 different medicinal preparations on the shelves in West Germany. According to a Slovakian folk saying, an individual should always bow when facing a chamomile plant — a sign of respect derived from hundreds of years experience with the folk medicine of that country.

Cinnamon
Cinnamomum zeylanicum

DESCRIPTION
Cinnamon is the dried, smooth inner bark of a cultivated laurel-like tree that grows in hot, wet tropical regions of India, Brazil, East and West Indies and Indian Ocean islands. The bark is sold in 2- to 18-inch (5 to 45 cm) lengths or "sticks," usually dried and rolled; cinnamon twigs (from *C. cassia*) are also used in Chinese medicine.

FLAVOR
Sweet, pungent.

PARTS USED
Bark.

HOW TO GROW
Type: a tropical tree native to Sri Lanka

HEALING PROPERTIES
Actions: carminative, diaphoretic, astringent, stimulant, antimicrobial

Uses: Cinnamon is a warming carminative used to promote digestion and relieve nausea, vomiting, and diarrhea. Its carminative, astringent and antimicrobial properties make it useful in upset stomach and Irritable Bowel Syndrome, and its additional warming properties for colds and flus. Recent research has shown that cinnamon helps the body use insulin more efficiently.

AVAILABILITY
Whole or cut, dried, rolled sticks available in supermarkets and alternative/health stores. Ground cinnamon and cinnamon powder widely available.

HOW TO USE IN COOKING
Cinnamon's spicy flavor blends well with apples and chocolate. Cinnamon is one of the spices in garam masala, an Indian blend used for savory dishes, rice and curries. It is usually used as a carminative with other herbs and spices. It may be used freely to flavor other herbal teas.
Whole sticks: used to flavor syrups, sauces, drinks and other liquids; usually removed after imparting flavor.
Crushed sticks: added to herbal spice and tea blends.
Powdered: used in sweet milk, cream and rice puddings and desserts; in cakes and biscuits, pastries, doughnuts and sweet fritters, mixed with brown or white sugar and sprinkled on porridge, cereal, coffee and toast; apple crisp and apple pies; pickles.

FOLKLORE
Chinese herbalists used cinnamon as far back as

2700 B.C., today they still recommend it for fever, diarrhea, and menstrual problems. Pliny, writing around AD 77 claimed, "...there is a tale of cinnamon growing around marshes under the protection of a terrible kind of bats...invented by the natives to raise the price." The ancient Egyptians used cinnamon in their embalming mixtures. India's ancient Ayurvedic healers used it to treat indigestion, as did the ancient Hebrews, Greeks, and Romans.

Clove
Syzygium aromaticum

DESCRIPTION
Pink, unopened flower buds of an evergreen tree native to Indonesia, now grown in Zanzibar, Madagascar, West Indies, Brazil, India and Sri Lanka. The nail-shaped buds turn red-brown when dried and are highly aromatic when dried.

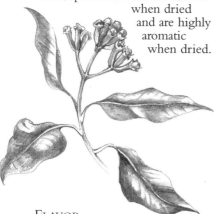

FLAVOR
Fragrantly strong, spicy taste.

PARTS USED
Dried buds.

HOW TO GROW
Type: A small, tropical evergreen tree, native to Southern Philippines

HEALING PROPERTIES
Actions: antioxidant, anesthetic, antiseptic, anti-inflammatory, anodyne, antispasmodic, carminative, stimulant, prevents vomiting, antihistamine, warming

Uses: Western herbalists use clove for nausea, vomiting, flatulence, diarrhea, hypothermia. Chinese physicians use it to treat indigestion, diarrhea, and intestinal parasites, as well as ringworm, athletes foot, and other fungal infections. Some studies indicate that cloves may have anticoagulant properties and stimulate the production of enzymes that fight cancer.

Phytochemistry: Cloves are the richest plant source of eugenol, which can boost antioxidant levels. Preliminary studies show that eugenol protects against cardiovascular disease by inhibiting the aggregation (abnormal clotting) of platelets. Some studies show that eugenol fights bacteria and inhibits the growth of many fungi, including *candida albicans*.
Clove oil, which is 60 to 90 percent eugenol, is the active ingredient in some mouthwashes, toothpastes, soaps, insect repellents, perfumes, foods, various veterinary medications and many over-the-counter toothache medications. Some dentists use clove oil as an oral anesthetic and to disinfect root canals.
Other sources of eugenol: allspice, bay rum, greater galangal, basil, nutmeg, turmeric, bay leaf, hyssop, oregano, marjoram

AVAILABILITY
Whole, dried buds and powder widely available.

HOW TO USE IN COOKING
Whole: in spiced or mulled wines, liqueurs; pickles; stocks, sauces and other liquids; studded in fruit and meats.
Ground: in sweet and savory sauces and glazes; to flavor apple and other fruit dishes; in curries, rice, soups and stews; mincemeat, traditional fruit puddings, cakes and stewed fruit dishes.

FOLKLORE
During the Han dynasty (207 BC to AD 220), the emperor required that everyone he addressed hold cloves in their mouths to mask bad breath. In Europe during the Middle Ages, they were widely used in cooking and as an antiseptic.

For toothache: Place a whole clove on the gum beside the ache, or between the teeth, nibbling at it until it has come to bits. Use no more than two cloves.

Dandelion
Taraxacum officinale

DESCRIPTION
A low-growing common plant that develops from a long, thick, dark brown tap root with white and milky flesh. Solitary, brilliant yellow round flowerhead sits atop a smooth, hollow stem. Oblong, bright green, deeply toothed leaves grow in a basal rosette directly from the root.

FLAVOR
Leaves are tart, bitter, somewhat chicory-like in taste; fresh root is nutty; roasted, dried root has a nutty, earthy flavor.

PARTS USED
Roots, stem, leaves, flowers.

HOW TO GROW
Type: hardy herbaceous perennial
Exposure: sun or shade; average soil
Propagation: from fresh seed; or transplant in spring, 18 inches (45 cm) apart; seed will self-sow; from sections of the root
Harvest: easily wildcrafted from organic fields; leaves and flowers in spring; dig root in the fall, store in a cool, dry place for 1 year

HEALING PROPERTIES
Actions:
Leaves: diuretic, liver and digestive tonic
Root: liver tonic, promotes bile flow, diuretic, mildly laxative, antirheumatic

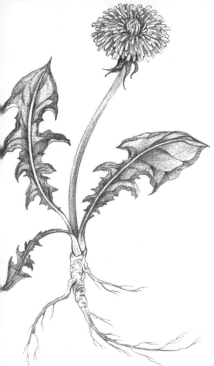

Dandelion is highest in lecithin (29,700 ppm) of any of the plant sources. Lecithin is important for cell membrane protection and replacement; reducing cholesterol; converting fat into energy; prevention of strokes and heart attacks and is used in Alzheimer's Disease.

Uses: Leaf is used specifically to support the kidney; the root, specifically to support the liver. Dandelion is used for liver, gall bladder, kidney, and bladder ailments, including hepatitis and jaundice; to promote the liver's processing of toxins for elimination; to provide important nutrients for storage or release into the system; in skin problems and rheumatism; and increases the flow of urine. As a diuretic, dandelion is important for its high potassium content since many other diuretics deplete the body's supply of potassium. Related disorders of digestion, such as dyspepsia, have also been shown to benefit from the ingestion of dandelion.

Phytochemistry: High in insulin, a form of carbohydrate easily assimilated by diabetics and hence is a potential source of nutritional support for diabetics.

Food value: dandelion is one of the best food sources of vitamin A

— *(greens per 100 g):* 187 mg calcium; 66 mg phosphorous; 3 mg iron; 397 mg potassium; 8,400 I.U. beta carotene; 35 mg vitamin C

AVAILABILITY

Whole plant easily foraged spring through fall. Fresh leaves in some supermarkets, farmers' markets, health/alternative stores; whole dried flowerheads in alternative/health stores; chopped, dried root in alternative/health stores.

HOW TO USE IN COOKING

Root: Fresh, peeled and cooked as any root vegetable or chopped in spring tonic; grated into salads. Dried root in tea, broths, soups, sauces, stews or any other long-simmering dish. Roasted roots are used as a coffee substitute, often blended with roasted chicory and/or burdock roots.
Leaf: Fresh, young, spring leaves used as a salad staple, steamed, braised, or sautéed as greens, with pasta, in soups and stocks.
Flower: Traditionally used for wine; fresh or dried to add color to sauces, butters, dips and cheese mixtures; in baked products, rice; chopped in salads, soups, egg dishes, custards and puddings; as a substitute for saffron; as a garnish for all main or dessert dishes; in cakes, breads and muffins; unopened buds steamed or sautéed with vegetables. Dried leaves and flowers are combined with other herbs such as nettles, burdock and yellow dock to make a herb beer or a healing tea blend.

FOLKLORE

The name comes from the French, *dent de Lion*, meaning that the leaves resemble lion's teeth. Arabian physicians of the 10th and 11th centuries seem to be the first to use dandelion as a medicine. In the 16th century, dandelion became known as *Herba urinaria* because of the

strong diuretic action of the leaves. This property is still reflected in both the English, (piss-a-bed) and French (*pissenlit*) common names.

Echinacea
(Purple Coneflower)
Echinacea angustifolia or *Echinacea purpurea*

DESCRIPTION

Deep purple petals seated around a high brown cone sit atop a 2- to 3-foot (60 to 90 cm) stem with ovate leaves that taper to a point at both ends. *Angustifolia* has thin leaves, *purpurea* has wider, more pointed leaves. Fragrant, tapering root is cylindrical, slightly spiral and tan in color.

FLAVOR

Root is sweet, pleasantly aromatic; flowers and stems are faintly aromatic.

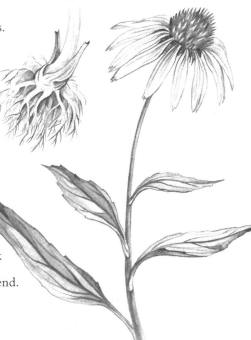

PARTS USED

Root is most powerful, but stems, leaves and petals of the plant may be used.

HOW TO GROW

Type: hardy perennial, native to North America
Exposure: full sun; average soil
Propagation: from seed or seedlings
Harvest: aerial parts in late summer while flowering; root after 2 to 3 seasons, in the fall, after the first frost

HEALING PROPERTIES

Actions: immune stimulating, anti-inflammatory, antibiotic, antimicrobial, antiseptic, analgesic, anti-allergenic, lymphatic tonic

Uses: Echinacea works best for illnesses that come and go and are not chronic. Studies have shown that it works best at the first sign of a cold or flu, taken in 4 to 6 doses daily for not more than 10 days.

One of the best herbs for overall health, clinical studies have confirmed traditional use of echinacea for boosting the immune system. German studies have shown that white blood cells stimulated by echinacea are up to 120% more effective in removing foreign bodies including bacteria and other pathogens from the blood stream. Taken at the early stages of a cold or flu, echinacea's phytochemical compounds stimulate white blood cells and lymphocytes to attack infected areas and destroy the invading organisms resulting in either a complete repulse of the attack or a shortened period of the cold or flu. Echinacea reduces the symptoms of inflammation. It has interferon-like actions, helping prevent and control viral infections. It hastens the healing of tissue by stimulating the fibroblasts that form new connective tissue. It fights viruses and *candida*. Finally, echinacea inhibits tumor growth — the result of a combination of all of the above actions.

AVAILABILITY

Whole or cut, dried root, and dried stems and leaves in alternative/health stores. Echinacea is also available in tincture and tablet form.

HOW TO USE IN COOKING

Using echinacea in cooking may aid in general well-being and help head off minor illnesses if taken in a soup for 2 or 3 days following bouts of stress or excessive fatigue. Echinacea combines well with garlic for healing colds and flus.
Petals and leaf: In salads, vegetable dishes, stir-fries, as garnish; in seasonings.
Root: Whole, fresh or dried, in long-simmering soups and stews; fresh grated into salads, vegetable dishes; ground, dried in spice blends, sauces, dips, puddings, desserts. Echinacea leaves, petals and finely chopped root, dried, blended with other herbs such as hyssop, peppermint and thyme can be used in teas as an effective cold remedy.
Tincture: Add 1 tsp (5 mL) to stocks, soups and stews when colds and flu threaten.

FOLKLORE

The Indian societies of the western plains and prairies used *E. angustifolia*, the narrow-leaved purple coneflower for more medicinal purposes (including snake bites, venomous insect bites and burns), than any other plant. Native Americans also used the fresh juice of echinacea to desensitize their feet before walking over hot coals during ceremonies and rituals.

To make echinacea tincture: In the fall, dig up one plant that is at least 3 years old. Wash flowers, leaves and stems and scrub root. Chop all parts to 1/2-inch (1 cm) pieces. Place into a large, wide-mouth jar. Cover with 80-proof drinking alcohol (vodka). Store in a cool, dark place for about 30 days, shaking the bottle every 3 to 4 days. Strain plant parts out and discard. Store tincture in smaller, brown or green bottles with tight-fitting lids, in cool, dark place. This makes enough tincture to last one family one or more years, depending on the use. Dose: 1/2 to 1 tsp (2 to 5 mL), 3 times daily for adults; double the dosage for best effect at the first sign of a cold, for a period of 1 day.

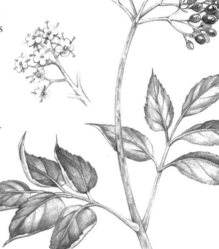

Elder
Sambucus nigra

DESCRIPTION

A medium-height (to 20 feet [6 m]) fast-growing shrub or small tree with flat-topped masses of creamy-white, fragrant blossoms which bear large drooping bunches of purplish-black berries. Dark green leaves are grouped in fives with finely serrated edges that taper to a point.

FLAVOR

Flowers are lightly aromatic; berries are tart and citrus tasting.

PARTS USED

Bark, flower and berries have the most medicinal value.

HOW TO GROW

Type: hardy perennial
Exposure: full sun; average soil
Propagation: from seed or seedlings
Harvest: flowers in the spring or early summer; berries in late summer; bark (from pruned limbs) in the fall

HEALING PROPERTIES

Actions:
Flowers: expectorant, reduces phlegm, circulatory, stimulant, promote sweating, diuretic, topically anti-inflammatory

Berries: promote sweating, diuretic, laxative
Bark: purgative, large doses promote vomiting, diuretic

Uses: Elderberry supports detoxification by promoting bowel movements, urination, sweating and secretion of mucus (for this reason, it is often found in commercially prepared cleansing products). Elderberry is effective in combating virus including colds and flu. Flu viruses have tiny spikes that cover their surfaces, which they use to invade human cells by puncturing the cell walls. These spikes are coated with an enzyme called neuraminidase, which helps break down the host cell's wall. The active ingredients in elderberries actually disarm the spikes by binding to them, coating them and preventing them from piercing the membrane. In addition, the elderberry's active components inhibit the action of the enzyme.
Elder flowers are taken early in the season to strengthen upper respiratory tract to help prevent hay fever.

Phytochemistry: Ripe berries are a good source of vitamins A, B, C and bioflavonoids.

Food value (elderberry per 100 g): 38 mg calcium; 28 mg phosphorus; 300 mg potassium; 360 I.U. beta carotene; 36 mg vitamin C.

AVAILABILITY
Dried flowers, fresh or dried berries available in alternative/ health stores.

HOW TO USE IN COOKING
Flowers: fresh, chopped into salads, lightly battered and fried; in wines, vinegars; syrups; dried in lemonade and other drinks.
Berries: fresh in jams, syrups, wines and jellies; blend with other fall fruits for desserts; vinegars, chutneys, ketchup. Dried berries (flavor improves on drying) and flowers are blended with other tea herbs. Elder syrups, jams and jellies may be used in hot or cold beverages, sauces and baked products.

FOLKLORE
Shakespeare calls it "the stinking Elder" in *Cymbeline* while referring to it as a symbol of grief. And in *Love's Labour Lost*, reference is made to the common mediaeval belief that "Judas was hanged on an Elder." The Holy Cross was believed to have been fashioned out of a giant elder tree. As a result of these stories and beliefs, elder became the symbol of sorrow and death. "In order to prevent witches from entering their houses, the common people used to gather Elder leaves on the last day of April and affix them to their doors and windows." — *Cole's Art of Simpling* (1656)

Garlic
Allium sativum

DESCRIPTION
The edible root is a bulb made up of 4 to 15 cloves enclosed in a white, tan or pinkish papery skin. Long (to 2 feet [60 cm]), flat, wide, grass-like leaves are sheathed at the base. At the tip of the round, hollow, sturdy stem, white flowers appear encased in a teardrop-like membrane that tapers to a sharp, green point. Flowers form a round ball when in full bloom.

FLAVOR
Hot, sharp, strong, unique taste.

PARTS USED
Bulb or "bud" at the root of the plant; scapes (the tall green stalks which form with immature flowerhead above ground); flowerhead

HOW TO GROW
Type: hardy perennial, thought to be native to Asia, possibly southern Siberia, but cultivated in the Mediterranean region for centuries
Exposure: full sun; dry, rich soil
Propagation: from seed or plant separated cloves 2 inches (5 cm) deep, 6 inches (15 cm) apart in late fall
Harvest: scapes in summer, before flowers open; bulbs in fall after stems have died back

HEALING PROPERTIES
Actions: anti-microbial, antibiotic, cardio-protective, hypotensive, anti-carcinogen, promotes sweating, reduces blood pressure, anti-coagulant, lowers blood cholesterol levels, lowers blood sugar levels, expectorant, digestive stimulant, diuretic, anti-histaminic, antiparasitic

Uses: Research has shown that garlic inhibits cancer cell formation and proliferation by inhibiting nitrosamine formation, modulating the metabolism of polyarene carcinogens, and by acting on cell enzymes which control cell division. Studies in Italy and China suggest that garlic consumption may offer a protective effect against gastric cancer (cancer of the stomach). Garlic lowers serum total and low density lipoprotein cholesterol in humans.

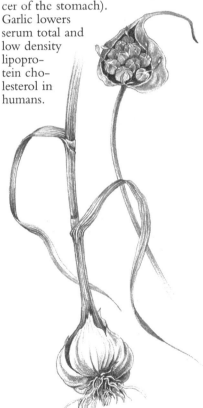

Studies in Spain and Italy, where the incidence of arteriosclerosis is low relative to other populations, have linked healthy arteries to a heavy consumption of garlic. Garlic reduces the tendency of the blood to clot, thereby reducing the risk of blocked arteries and heart disease.

Five studies of patients with high total serum cholesterol levels showed that eating about half a clove of garlic per day can decrease TSC levels by about 9%. Garlic also raises high density lipoprotein cholesterol (HDLs) in humans.

Garlic offers strong antioxidant protection to cell membranes against free radical formation. Some studies show that even in low doses, garlic stimulates the immune system, increasing the activity of natural "killer cells" to ward off pathogens.

Garlic has strong antibiotic properties; it kills intestinal parasites and worms, as well as gram-negative bacteria. In recent studies, researchers using fresh and powdered garlic solutions discovered that garlic inhibited many bacteria including *staphylococcus auras, E coli, proteus vulgaris, salmonella enteritidis, Klebsiella pneumonia* and many others.

And, when compared to antibiotics such as penicillin, tetracyclines, erytromycin and other commonly prescribed antibiotics, garlic proved to be as effective. One medium-sized garlic clove delivers the antibacterial equivalent of about 100,000 units of penicillin (typical oral penicillin doses range from 600,000 to 1.2 million units, equivalent to 6 to 12 cloves of garlic).

Garlic inhibits inflammation, which makes it, in conjunction with its antibacterial properties, to be a good wound medicine. Garlic protects organs — the liver from damage induced by synthetic drugs and chemical pollutants, and in addition, protects against the effects of radiation.

Garlic lowers blood pressure. Many studies indicate that garlic may lower both systolic and diastolic blood pressure in hypertensives.

Phytochemistry: Allicin found in cut, cooked, or otherwise processed garlic, is one of the plant kingdom's most potent, broad-spectrum antibiotics (it destroys *candida albicans*). Adenosine lowers blood pressure; Ajoene prevents blood clots and is believed to be at least as strong as aspirin as an anticoagulant; diallyl sulfides, phenolic acid and quercetin fight carcinogens and lower cholesterol. Selenium and germanium are anti-cancer compounds.

Organosulphur compounds derived from garlic inhibit experimental mutagenesis. Fresh garlic contains more organosulphides, weight for weight, than even the most expensive 'medicinal' extracts.

Food value (1 clove, raw): 6 g protein; 29 mg calcium; 202 mg phosphorus; 529 mg potassium; 15 mg vitamin C.

AVAILABILITY

Fresh whole bulbs at farmers' markets, food stores and supermarkets; scapes at Chinese and some farmers' markets.

HOW TO USE IN COOKING

Most research has been based on epidemiological studies of populations that have a high consumption of garlic in whole food form. This gives us reason to believe that cooking with garlic and eating it fresh, often raw, every day will give us the same benefits. To get reliable medicinal benefit from garlic, it is recommended that about two medium-sized whole garlic bulbs or buds be taken per week (about 2 oz [50 g]). That requires that almost every main dish you consume contain a minimum of two cloves each. Start to increase your fresh garlic consumption by blending minced fresh garlic into prepared sauces, dips and salad dressings. For every clove called for in recipes (other than those in this book), always use 2 to 3. Dried, powdered garlic has no medicinal qualities.

Tip: chew fresh parsley to mask garlic's odor on the breath.

Bud: whole, roasted to caramelize the sugars for use in spreads, dips, sauces

Cloves: whole as a mild seasoning rub for meats, salad bowls and roasted for sauces, vegetable & pasta dishes; whole, blanched (boiled 30 seconds in water) to add subtle flavor to dressings or stir-fries; puréed blanched cloves used to thicken sauces; half cloves added to spiced oils and vinegars; slivers in stir-fries, rice dishes; chopped, fresh, raw cloves in salad dressings, aioli, pestos, hummus, salsas; cooked in all main dishes and sauces.

Scapes: fresh, chopped into dips, salads, sauces, salad dressing, as a garnish; stir-fried with butter and lemon or added to grilled or baked vegetable and rice dishes

Flower: as a garnish; in vinegars and oils; chopped in salads, stir-fries and other main dishes.

FOLKLORE

Mohammedan legend holds that, "when Satan stepped out from the Garden of Eden after the fall of man, Garlick sprang up from the spot where he placed his left foot, and Onion from that where his right foot touched."

In Homer's *Odyssey*, Ulysses turns to garlic for strength against the sorceress Circe. Shakespeare called it the "stinking rose," Romans ate it for strength in battle, Egyptian slaves ate it as they built the pyramids and doctors used garlic in World War I to disinfect wounds (the raw juice was diluted with water, and applied to wounds on swabs of sterilized sphagnum moss).

GARLIC SYRUP

Syrup of Garlic was once thought of as a remedy for asthma.

12	cloves garlic, minced or crushed	12
1 cup	boiling water	250 mL
2 tbsp	apple cider vinegar	25 mL
1/4 cup	honey	50 mL

1. Put garlic in a clean jar; pour water over and cover with lid. Keep in a cool place for 10 to 12 hours, shaking the jar occasionally.

2. Strain water into a small bowl, pressing on garlic to remove as much liquid as possible (discard garlic). Stir vinegar and honey into garlic water, pour into clean jar with tight-fitting lid.

Dose: 1 tbsp (15 mL) 3 times per day as an expectorant

Makes: 1 1/2 cups (375 mL)

Store: in refrigerator, up to 3 months. Grieve gives this remedy for asthma, "syrup of Garlic, made by boiling the bulbs till soft and adding an equal quantity of vinegar to the water in which they have been boiled, and then sugared and boiled down to a syrup. The syrup is then poured over the boiled bulbs, which have been allowed to dry meanwhile, and kept in a jar. Each morning a bulb or two is to be taken, with a spoonful of the syrup."[4]

Ginger
Zingiber officinale

DESCRIPTION

Erect reed-like stems grow from the aromatic, light tan colored, thick, fleshy, scaly rhizomes which branch with thick, thumb like protrusions. Yellow-green flowers, tinged with purple, grow in dense, cone-like spikes. Narrow, sword-shaped leaves grow from the 2- to 4-foot (60 to 120 cm) reed-like stem.

HOW TO GROW

Type: tender perennial, native to Southeast Asia
Exposure: Full sun; warm, moist, sheltered location
Propagation: from root cuttings
Harvesting: Harvest after 2 or 3 years' growth. Dig roots in the fall after the tops have died back. Store in a cool, dark, dry place or keep in the freezer.

FLAVOR

Fresh: hot, sweet, spicy-citrus, biting
Dried: powdered has a stronger, more bitter taste

PARTS USED

Root.

HEALING PROPERTIES

Actions: anti-nausea, relieves headaches and arthritis, anti-inflammatory, circulatory stimulant, expectorant, antispasmodic, antiseptic, diaphoretic, guards against blood clots, peripheral

vasodilator, prevents vomiting, carminative, antioxidant

Uses:
Ginger root calms nausea and prevents vomiting. In tests for motion sickness, ginger proved more effective than Dramamine® in preventing motion sickness, as reported by the medical journal *Lancet.* Later studies found ginger to be highly effective against the most severe form of morning sickness, *hyperemesis gravidarum.* Ginger may also alleviate nausea caused by drug therapy including highly toxic chemotherapy drugs.
Ginger root is a cleansing herb. It has a warming effect and supports digestion while stimulating circulation and sweating. Ginger contains powerful enzymes and increases the action of the gall bladder, while protecting the liver against toxins.
Ginger reduces total volume of acid in the stomach and prevents the formation of ulcers from a wide variety of causes including stress, alcohol and other stomach irritants.
Ginger extract inhibits platelet aggregation, the key factor in the formation of blood clots, which can help prevent heart attack and stroke. It also helps lower blood cholesterol and strengthen the heart muscle. Based on research results, an outpatient cardiology clinic in Israel now recommends that all of its patients take 1/2 tsp (2 mL) powdered ginger daily.
Studies show ginger giving some relief from the pain and swelling of arthritis without side effects.
An ingredient of as many as half of all herbal prescriptions in China, ginger is believed to decrease the toxicity of other ingredients.

Phytochemistry: Gingerol is one of ginger's pungent principle constituents.

CAUTION

Ginger can be irritating to the intestinal mucosa, and should be taken with or after meals. Ginger is contraindicated in kidney disease.

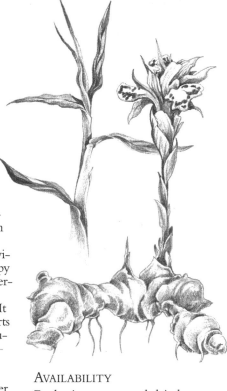

AVAILABILITY

Fresh ginger root and dried powdered ginger is widely available in supermarkets, Asian and Indian markets and health/alternative stores. Dried, candied and candied ginger in syrup is available in some supermarkets and specialty stores.

HOW TO USE IN COOKING

Gingerols, present in the fresh rhizome, convert into the more pungent shogaols when subjected to dehydration and heat. Both of these constituents possess therapeutic properties, so you should use fresh or dried, ground ginger liberally in cooking as a general tonic (hormone balancer) and to ward off colds and flu. Cook with fresh and dried ginger daily if you or someone in your family suffers from migraine headaches, if influenza threatens, if rheumatoid arthritis is diagnosed, if joint stiffness is a problem, or if embarking on a weight loss program.
Fresh: sliced to flavor vinegars, oils or stocks; julienned in stir-fries; chopped or grated, raw in salad dressings, marinades; chopped, cooked in all main dishes, stir-fries, cakes, baked goods, preserves and pickles; juice to flavor salad dressings, marinades or sauces; candied in fruit salads, desserts, salad dress-

ings and sauces. Peel and chop fresh ginger, allow to dry and blend with other herbs for teas.
To store fresh root: in a cool, dry place for several days; wrap in a paper towel and set in an open plastic bag to keep for several weeks in the refrigerator; seal fresh root in plastic bag, freeze and cut off as needed or peel and slice, place in a glass jar, cover with vodka, seal and refrigerate (keeps indefinitely).
Candied dry and Candied in syrup: the hot flavor of ginger is mitigated by the sugar. Use where fresh ginger is called for, especially in desserts and drinks. Candied ginger keeps for a year or longer, and is easy to use in cooking. (See page 40 for information on making candied roots.)
Leaves: as a decorative plate liner, to wrap fish for the grill, or to serve finger foods and hors d'oeuvres.
Flowers: if available, use for salads and as an edible garnish.
Dried: powdered in cooking as you would fresh. Take 1/3 tsp (1 mL) in water every 3 to 4 hours to relieve nausea, motion sickness.

To make ginger tea: Place 5 or 6 thin slices of ginger root (or 1/2 tsp [2 mL] dried) in a non-metallic teapot. Pour 1 cup (250 mL) boiling water over and place lid on pot. Steep for 30 minutes. For a stronger tea, simmer gently for 10 to 15 minutes.

FOLKLORE

Our gingerbread may have evolved from the Greek tradition of eating ginger wrapped in bread after meals in order to help with digestion. Ginger was recognized by Ayurvedic medicine as "the universal remedy."
For centuries, Japanese people have been serving pickled and other forms of ginger with sushi and other raw fish dishes.
Modern science has now proven that ginger is effective against parasites, including those found in uncooked fish such as the protozoan anisakis, the most common parasitic infection in Japan. Our modern soft drink, ginger ale (a derivative of 17th-century ginger beer), is still a good aid for mild stomach upset and/or nausea.

Ginseng

Siberian *(Eleutherococcus senticosis),* North American *(Panax quinquefolius)* and Asian *(Panax ginseng)*

DESCRIPTION

Large, fleshy, light yellow or tan colored, slow-growing root, 2 to 3 inches (5 to 7.5 cm) in length and from 1/2 to 1 inch (1 to 2.5 cm) around, out of which grows a foothigh (30 cm) stem. Three stems, each with 5 ovate leaves, grow out of the top of the stem, bright red berries appear in late summer.

FLAVOR

Bitter sweet, earthy, sometimes musky flavor.

PARTS USED

Fresh or dried root from mature (over 4 years old) plants, when available and if organic, spring leaves.

HOW TO GROW

Type: hardy perennial, native to cool, wooded area of eastern and central North America
Exposure: 80% shade; loose, fertile, well-drained soil with a heavy mulch of leaves
Propagation: root cuttings, or from seed

Harvesting: after 4 years' growth, dig roots in the fall after the tops have died back. Store in a cool, dark, dry place.

HEALING PROPERTIES

Actions: antioxidant, adaptogen, tonic, stimulant, regulates blood sugar and cholesterol levels, stimulates the immune system

Uses: Ginseng helps the body better resist and adapt to stress. It is a mild stimulant and as a tonic, it pro-

motes long-term overall health. Along with increasing resistance to diabetes, cancer, heart disease, and various infections, the medical literature on ginseng claims that it can improve memory, increase fertility, protect the liver against many toxins, and protect the body from radiation. Traditional Chinese medicine uses Asian ginseng to revitalize and as a tonic during times of fatigue, reduced work capacity and concentration, and during convalescence. American ginseng is used to cool and soothe, quench thirst, and reduce fevers.

Phytochemistry: The active chemicals in ginseng are called ginsenosides, and occur nowhere else in nature. Several ginsenosides either stimulate or depress the activity of the central nervous system, many of which are known to have specific effects on the immune, hormonal, cardiovascular, and central nervous systems. Many other ginsenosides are antioxidant compounds.

CAUTION

As a rule, avoid ginseng if you have a fever, asthma, bronchitis, emphysema, high blood pressure, or cardiac arrhythmia. Avoid in pregnancy, with hyperactivity in children, or taken with coffee.

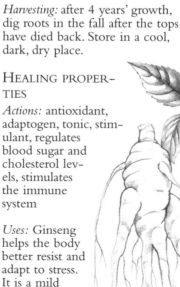

AVAILABILITY

Dried root (whole or chopped), tea, and powder are all found in health/alternative stores and Asian grocery stores. Dried leaf sometimes found in health/alternative stores and direct from chemical-free growers.

HOW TO USE IN COOKING

To preserve fresh ginseng roots, they are sometimes steamed and fried, becoming more potent. When prepared this way, they take on a reddish color, and are known as "red ginseng."

Cooked in dishes, ginseng imparts only a slight flavor to the food. Use in the same way as ginger.

Dried ginseng is very hard and brittle. A good grater, like those used for nutmeg will shred the root fine.

Whole: fresh or dried in soups, stocks and stews.

Dried flakes: used in long-simmering soups and stews, then strained off.

Chopped: fresh or dried, in muesli and grain-nut-fruit energy bars; in whole grain toppings for desserts; mixed with other herbs for tea blends.

Ground dried: in milkshakes and smoothies; salad dressings; in puddings and other cooked desserts; as part of an antibiotic herbal seasoning, chili pastes, *roux* and to flavor honey.

Leaves: use only if organic; dried, brewed into teas, then added to soups, broths, stews, puddings.

FOLKLORE

The word ginseng is said to mean "the wonder of the world," the generic name, panax, comes from the Greek *panakos* (panacea) which describes how the Chinese regarded it — the essence of the earth in condensed form. Both the American Indian name, *garantoquen,* and the Chinese, *jin-chen,* have the same meaning — "like a man" — referring to the resemblance of the roots to the human form. Canadian Jesuits began harvesting wild ginseng and shipping the roots to China in 1718 and their export became second only to fur in importance. Within the last decade, Canadian commercial production of ginseng has grown to over 1 million pounds (500,000 kg) annually, with about 90 percent of that amount being exported to China.

Green Tea
Camellia sinensis

DESCRIPTION

Green and black tea comes from the shrub or small tree indigenous to the wet forests of Asia and cultivated commercially in Asia, Africa, South America, and North Carolina. To produce green tea, whole or rolled leaves are steamed or heated (removing the oxidizing enzyme that turns the leaves black), then dried. Black tea is produced by rolling the leaves, exposing them to air (thus promoting oxidation of polyphenols) in a fermentation process, then drying by warm air.

FLAVOR
Bitter-sweet.

PARTS USED
Leaves.

HOW TO GROW
A tropical tree, native to India and Asia.

HEALING PROPERTIES

Actions: antioxidant, stimulant, astringent, antibacterial, diuretic, anti-tumor, anti-obesity, prevents gum disease and cavities, lowers blood pressure and blood sugar levels, lowers cholesterol

Uses: Green tea is a good tonic beverage and can be mixed with other herbs for teas. Early studies have shown anti-cancer effects and its efficacy in preventing heart disease, lowering blood pressure, regulating blood sugar levels, warding off colds and flu, and preventing gum disease and cavities. Epidemiological studies of Japanese people, heavy consumers of green tea, show that they have lower death rates from cancer of all types, especially cancer of the stomach.

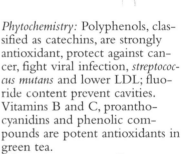

Phytochemistry: Polyphenols, classified as catechins, are strongly antioxidant, protect against cancer, fight viral infection, *streptococcus mutans* and lower LDL; fluoride content prevent cavities. Vitamins B and C, proanthocyanidins and phenolic compounds are potent antioxidants in green tea.

All teas have some caffeine: black teas, 4 to 4.5 percent; green and oolong teas, 3 to 4 percent — about one-quarter to one-third the caffeine in coffee.

AVAILABILITY

Dried, bulk in Oriental markets and alternative/health stores; individually wrapped in supermarkets

Types of Japanese green tea available:

Mat-cha: intense flavor, best quality, highest price, used for the tea ceremony

Sen-cha: sweet-bitter taste, medium-grade

Ban-cha: astringent, most common type of green tea available

Genmai-cha: mild, nutty flavor, mixture of roasted rice and *Ban-cha*

Hoji-cha: smokey flavor, lightly roasted *Ban-cha*

Kuki-cha: earthy flavor, made of stems and twigs

HOW TO USE IN COOKING

Use green tea for syrups, dressings and puddings. Blend dried green tea with other dried herbs for a beverage.
To make green tea: Use 1 tbsp (15 mL) tea and 1 cup (250 mL) boiling water per person. Steep tea only 30 seconds before serving.

FOLKLORE

In Japan, the Buddhist monk who attended and cured the ailing Shogun Sanetomo with green tea is credited with reintroducing green tea to Japan. It is believed that Zen Buddhist monks designed the 500-year-old Japanese tea ceremony, now a part of their cultural heritage. Tea was introduced to the English court in the dowry of the young Portuguese bride of King Charles II in the 1660s.

Hyssop
Hyssopus officinalis

DESCRIPTION

An evergreen, bushy, woody plant that grows to 1 or 2 feet (30 to 60 cm). The square, upright stem bears linear, opposite leaves and purple flowers in whorls from the dense spikes at the top of the stems.

FLAVOR

Minty, peppery, slightly bitter, pungent.

PARTS USED

Leaves and flowering tops.

HOW TO GROW

Type: hardy perennial, native to central and southern Europe, naturalized in North America
Exposure: full sun; light, well-drained soil
Propagation: from seed, tip cuttings or by division
Harvest: aerial parts in summer when flowering

HEALING PROPERTIES

Actions: expectorant, carminative, relaxes peripheral blood vessels, promotes sweating, reduces phlegm, antiviral (*herpes simplex*), antispasmodic

Uses: Hyssop's antispasmodic and expectorant properties make it useful in coughs, bronchitis and sore throats. As a diaphoretic and sedative, it is useful in colds, flu and children's fevers. Hyssop also helps with fevers. New research points to it as an anti-HIV agent. It is also applied on the skin to help reduce inflammation and heal bruises and ulcers.

Phytochemistry: Caffeic acid and unspecified tannins in extracts of hyssop have been shown to have strong anti-HIV activity.

AVAILABILITY

Whole/cut dried leaves and flowers available in alternative/health stores.

HOW TO USE IN COOKING

The green tops, boiled in soup, have actually been used in the treatment of asthma.
Leaves and flowers: fresh, in salads, fruit cocktails and wraps; fresh or dried leaves and/or flowers in baked goods (especially brownies and date squares), fruit flans and pies, dessert and cough syrups, jams, jellies, sauces, dessert dishes, soups, stews, stock, stuffings and particularly with pork and fatty

fish (hyssop has grease-cutting qualities); dried and mixed with green tea and other herbs for beverages.

FOLKLORE

Hyssop's essential oil, distilled from the leaves, stems and flowers, has a highly aromatic odor and this made it more prized by perfumers than oil of lavender. The earliest recorded use of the plant was as a strewing herb to cleanse the air in sickrooms — in the "language of flowers," hyssop symbolizes cleanliness and sacrifice.
Hyssop is a bee plant, legend telling of beekeepers who rubbed their hives with it to entice bees to stay.

Lavender
Lavendula
English (*Lavendula angustifolia*), French (*Lavendula dentata*), among many species

DESCRIPTION

A woody, shrub-like plant (grows to 3 feet [90 cm] in hot, dry areas), with dense, woody stems from which linear, pine-like, grey-green leaves grow. The flowers grow in spikes from young shoots, on long stems. The spikes are composed of whorls of tiny flowers, each composed of from 6 to 10 flowers.

FLAVOR

Fragrant, perfumy.

PARTS USED

Leaves and flowers.

HOW TO GROW

Type: perennial, English is hardy to zone 2; French is better adapted to zone 5, native to the Mediterranean
Exposure: full sun; light, sandy, well-drained soil; protected
Propagation: seedlings planted in spring; cuttings or root division
Harvesting: Harvest leaves and flowers toward the end of flowering, in the morning or early evening, when the essential oils in the flowers are at their height

HEALING PROPERTIES

Actions: antispasmodic, circulatory stimulant, relaxant, tonic for the nervous system, antibacterial, analgesic, carminative, promotes bile flow, antiseptic

Uses: Lavender is used as a relaxant for stress-related headaches and in promoting sleep. As a circulatory stimulant, it can be applied externally to relieve the pains of arthritis. Lavender is also used in creams and salves to heal wounds.

Phytochemistry: Laboratory research on the anti-cancer activity of perillyl alcohol, distilled from lavender shows promise in the fight against cancer of the breast, pancreas, colon, and prostate.

AVAILABILITY

Dried leaves and flowers available in alternative/health stores.

HOW TO USE IN COOKING

Flower: fresh or dried, in baked goods such as cookies, cakes, scones, quick breads, sauces, jellies, sorbets, vinegars; in deglazed pan juices from sautéed lamb, pork or chicken; as a garnish; to flavor honey and vinegar; in jams, jellies and candies. Dried flowers and leaves in herbes de Provence spice blend and in

sugar substitutes; blended with other herbs and green tea. Lavender teams nicely with lemon in tarts and other desserts and was used to flavor condiments. Gerard speaks of Conserves of Lavender being served at table.

FOLKLORE

Indigenous to the mountainous regions of the countries bordering the western half of the Mediterranean, lavender was not cultivated in England until 1568 and was one of the plants which the Pilgrim Fathers took to the new world.

To make toilette vinegar:

1/2 cup	dried rose leaves	125 mL
1/2 cup	lavender flowers	125 mL
2 cups	white vinegar	500 mL
1 cup	rosewater	250 mL

Put dried leaves and flowers in a jar with a tight-fitting lid. Pour vinegar over, cap and allow to stand in the sun for 2 to 3 days. Strain and mix aromatic vinegar with rosewater, shake well and pour into smaller bottles. Splash over neck and arms or use with a spritz for a refreshing spray all day long. Makes 3 cups (750 mL).

Licorice
Glycyrrhiza
European *(glycyrrhiza glabra)* and Chinese *(glycyrrhiza uralensis)* are the species available in the North American market for medicinal use.

DESCRIPTION

Licorice sticks are 6- to 8-inch (15 to 20 cm) segments of the underground stems (stolons) of the plant which may extend as far as 20 feet (6 m) from the main root. Wrinkled and brown on the outside, licorice root is yellow on the inside.
The 3- to 6-foot (90 to 180 cm) plants are hairy Eurasian herbs of the pea family *(leguminosae),* with compound leaves,

pea like flowers, and leathery or prickly inflated pods.

PARTS USED

Whole root (extracts lack the tonic action), powdered root.

HOW TO GROW

Type: tender perennial, hardy in zones 7 to 9, native to Mediterranean region and southwest Asia
Exposure: full sun; sandy soil, near streams or in river valleys
Propagation: easily grown from divisions or root cuttings planted 1 to 1 1/2 inches (2.5 to 4 cm) apart, or sow seeds outdoors in spring or fall
Harvesting: Harvest after 3 or 4 year's growth. Dig roots in the fall after the tops are dry. Scrub clean, dry the roots for several months, then store in a cool place.

FLAVOR

Sweet, earthy flavor — although we think of licorice as a flavor, the taste most people associate with licorice is actually anise — the terms anise and licorice are now commonly interchangeable; however, the medicinal qualities are not. Licorice root is 50 times as sweet as table sugar.

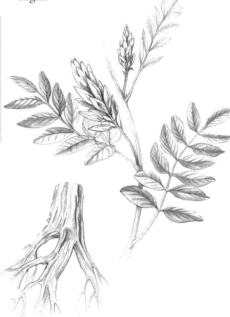

HEALING PROPERTIES

Actions: biochemical balancer, gentle laxative, tonic, anti-inflammatory, antibacterial, anti-arthritic, lowers blood cholesterol, soothes gastric mucous membranes, expectorant

Uses: Licorice root is considered one of the best tonic herbs because it provides nutrients to almost all body systems. It detoxifies, helping to eliminate poisons and toxins from the body (it is taken to protect the liver), regulates blood sugar levels and recharges depleted adrenal glands and combats allergies.

It powerfully supports the adrenal glands in their roles of reducing inflammation and stimulating tissue repair and growth. It has also been shown to heal stomach ulcers and is used to soothe irritated membranes and loosen and expel phlegm in the upper respiratory tract.

It is used to treat sore throat, urinary tract infections, and constipation. In Chinese medicine, herbs are designated as either "monarch," "minister," "assistant," or "guide." Licorice is a guide herb in half of all Chinese prescriptions. Guide herbs enhance the effects of the other ingredients, reduce toxicity and improve taste.

Phytochemistry: Glycoside glycyrrhizin (or glycyrrhizic acid), 50 to 150 times sweeter than sucrose, is the plant's major active constituent. It encourages the production of hormones such as hydrocortisone.

CAUTION

Eating large amounts of licorice can produce headaches, water retention and imbalances of sodium and potassium. German health authorities warn that it should not be used for more than 4 to 6 weeks in therapeutic doses except on medical advice. Licorice should not be used at all if you are pregnant, have high blood pressure, potassium deficiency in the blood, or chronic inflammation or cirrhosis of the liver.

AVAILABILITY

Whole or powdered, dried root available at alternative/health food stores.

HOW TO USE IN COOKING

Licorice is used by brewers — it gives port and stout their characteristic black color and thick consistency. It can also be used in cooking for the same purpose in sauces, puddings and gravies. Make a tea by simmering 1 teaspoon of the cut and sifted dried root in a cup of boiling water for 5 minutes. Strain the tea and use for sauces, in baked goods such as cookies, and puddings.

FOLKLORE

Dioscorides named the plant Glyrrhiza from the Greek *glukos* for sweet and *riza*, a root. It appears that licorice extract was in common use in Germany during the Middle Ages. King Edward I of England taxed licorice imports in 1305 to finance repairs of London Bridge. Napoleon chewed licorice sticks, which are said to have turned his teeth black. Native North Americans and early European settlers used the native *G. lepidota* to bring on menstrual periods, expel the placenta following childbirth, and relieve earache, toothache, and fever.

In England, a commercial lozenge called Pontefract or Pomfrey cakes is made from extract of licorice from home-grown roots. Pontefract cakes date from the 18th century, when chemist George Dunhill of Pontefract, England began to make the sweets from licorice root extract, molasses, sugar, and flour.

To make extract of licorice:

2	6-inch (15 cm) sticks licorice, crushed	2
2 cup	water	500 mL

1. In a non-reactive saucepan, bring licorice and water to a boil, reduce heat slightly and keep simmering gently until mixture thickens slightly, about 40 to 60 minutes.

2. Allow to cool completely, then strain and pour into a clean bottle. Store in refrigerator for up to one month. Makes 2 cups (500 mL) extract.

Mushrooms
Shiitake mushroom *(lentinula edodes)*, Maitake mushroom *(grifola frondosa)*

DESCRIPTION

According to Grieve, fungi are "those plants which are colorless...having no chlorophyll, fungi cannot use the energy of the sun and must therefore adopt another method of life. They either live as parasites on other living plants or animals, or they live on decaying matter."[5]

Shiitake: amber to brown cap, traditional mushroom shape, medium in size

Maitake: means "dancing mushroom" in Japan because it is made up of many overlapping, fan-shaped fruit bodies that resemble butterflies dancing. Called "hen of the woods" in North America because it grows in big clusters resembling a hen's tail feathers, at the base of trees or stumps.

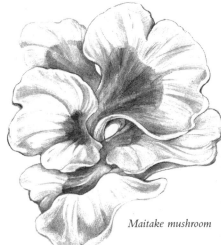

Maitake mushroom

FLAVOR
Delicious, earthy, nutty taste.

---

5. *Ibid,* Vol. II, p. 331

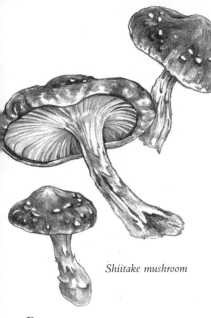

Shiitake mushroom

PARTS USED
Mushroom cap and stem.

HOW TO GROW
Type: fungus
Exposure: mottled shade
Propagation: from spores

HEALING PROPERTIES (SHIITAKE)
Actions: immune-boosting, anti-tumor, anti-cancer, anti-viral, anti-AIDS, antibacterial, cholesterol lowering, hepatoprotective and liver-protective properties

Uses: Strengthened immune response from shiitake mushrooms means increased body resistance to bacterial, viral, fungal, and parasitic infections. Shiitake is beneficial for soothing bronchial inflammation, regulating urinary incontinence, reducing chronic high cholesterol, and inhibiting cancer metastasis. It is used in arthritis and chronic fatigue syndrome.

Phytochemistry: Lenitnan in shiitake mushrooms has been shown to enhance immunity cells in clearing the body of tumor cells and in fighting HIV and hepatitis B viruses. Lentinan is one of three different anti-cancer drugs extracted from mushrooms approved by Japan's Health and Welfare Ministry.

Food Value: Shiitake mushrooms are high in vitamin C and calcium and zinc.

HEALING PROPERTIES (MAITAKE)
Actions: hepatoprotective, antihypotensive, anti-breast cancer and colorectal cancer

Uses: In the late 1980s, Japanese scientists identified the maitake as being more potent than any mushroom previously studied. Maitake has remarkable tonic effects, especially on the immune system. It is used in the prevention of some cancers and may help protect against high blood pressure, constipation, diabetes, and HIV.

Phytochemistry: Maitake's polysaccharide compound, known as beta 1,6 glucan (or D-fraction) is recognized by researchers as the most effective active agent stimulating cellular immune responses and inhibiting tumors.

CAUTION
Raw mushrooms contain hydrazines, potentially toxic substances which are destroyed in cooking or drying. Do not use fresh, raw mushrooms; always cook them.

AVAILABILITY
Whole fresh available in Oriental markets, alternative/health stores, and some supermarkets. Whole or cut, dried available in Oriental markets, alternative/health stores and some supermarkets.

HOW TO USE IN COOKING
To get the amount you would need for medicinal doses, you would have to eat 3.5 oz (90 g) per day, which might cause stomach upset. However, cooking with shiitake and maitake mushrooms at least three times per week (more if possible) will contribute to overall immune and cardiovascular health and will lower your risk of cancer. According to Dr. Moss, an expert in cancer treatment, incorporating fresh or dried shiitake into a diet rich in whole grains, vegetables and fruits is a low-cost cancer prevention strategy.[6]

Fresh: whole, roasted or grilled; halved, in stews, soups; sliced in rice (risotto) and grain dishes, stir-fries, roasted vegetable dishes; shredded raw in salads, sandwiches.

Dried: add to soups and stews; reconstitute by soaking in water, then use as suggested above, saving and using the soaking water for soups, stews, gravies, sauces and to add to other cooking liquids.

FOLKLORE
The ancient Chinese believed that shiitake dispelled hunger, treated colds, and nourished the circulatory system. In the 14th century, Chinese physician Wu Rui described shiitake as a food that activates qi (the life force). The 6th International Mycological Congress coined the phrase "bioremediation of toxins," referring to the unique ability of medicinal mushrooms to seek out and absorb systemic toxins for elimination.

Parsley
Petroselinum crispum
(curled leaf parsley)

DESCRIPTION
Branching stems support bright green leaves divided into feather-like sections. Leaves lie flat or curl into frilly leaflets, depending on the variety. Flowers appear in the second year, in umbels.

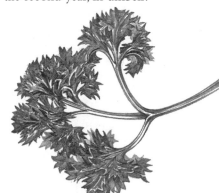

[6.] "Promising Alternative Treatments for Cancer," by Sibylle Preuschat, *Health Naturally* magazine, April/May 1996, p. 32; reprinted with permission.

HOW TO GROW

Type: hardy biennial, grown as an annual in colder climates, native to the Mediterranean
Exposure: part shade; rich, moist soil
Propagation: from seed (slow germinating), thin to 8 inches (20 cm) apart; or nursery plants
Harvesting: harvest all season

FLAVOR

Leaves have a tangy-sweet, "green" taste; root is faintly aromatic with a sweet taste.

PARTS USED

Leaves, stems and roots.

HEALING PROPERTIES

Actions: antioxidant, tonic, digestive, diuretic

Uses: As a diuretic, it helps the body get rid of excess water (flushes the kidneys), and is often used in rheumatism. As a nutrient, it is one of the richest food sources of vitamin C. It is commonly eaten to dispel garlic's odor.

Phytochemistry: An excellent source of vitamins A and C , iron, and at least two antioxidants — beta-carotene and lutein. Chlorophyll and myristicin may also inhibit the development of some cancers.

Food value (fresh, per 100 g): 390 mg calcium; 200 mg phosphorus; 17.9 mg iron; 3,200 I.U. beta carotene; 281 mg vitamin C; *(dried, per 100 g):* 351 g phosphorus; 97.9 mg iron; 3,805 mg potassium; 23,340 I.U. beta carotene; 7.9 mg miacin; 122 mg vitamin C.

CAUTION

Should not be used in high doses during pregnancy as this may cause excessive uterine stimulation. Parsley's high concentration of oxalates makes calcium inaccessible to the body and people with osteoporosis should limit their intake. It is contraindicated in kidney inflammation because, as a diuretic, it provides too much stimulation for kidneys that are in need of rest.

AVAILABILITY

Fresh sprigs in most supermarkets year-round.

HOW TO USE IN COOKING

Fresh parsley can be used in almost any dish as it blends well with other flavors.
Whole sprigs: for background flavoring for soups, stews, vegetable or fish poaching water; with other herbs as a stuffing for fish and poultry.
Leaves: fresh, torn in sandwiches, salads, chopped in spreads, vegetable (especially peas and potatoes) and grain salads; fresh or dried in casseroles, soups, stuffings, sausages, tomato, fish or egg dishes; finely chopped as a garnish for noodles, vegetables, casseroles. *Persillade* is a fine mince of garlic and parsley added at the last to sautés, grilled dishes and casseroles, lentils and vegetables, especially steamed peas and potatoes. *Fines herbes* is a seasoning blend of equal parts: parsley, chives, tarragon, basil and thyme.
Root: boil the fresh root and serve as parsnip or add to soups, stocks and stews.

FOLKLORE

Gerard claims, "It is delightful to the taste and agreeable to the stomache...the roots or seeds boiled in ale and drank, cast foorth strong venome or poyson; but the seed is the strongest part of the herbe." Wreaths of parsley adorned graves and took root and flourished, causing it to be associated with death, the underworld and ill fortune. A common expression, "to be in need of parsley," referred to one who was hopelessly ill.

Peppermint
Mentha piperita

DESCRIPTION

Square, purple stems grow 2 to 4 feet (60 to 120 cm) with bright green, oval, toothed leaves with pointed tips growing opposite. Small pink, white or purple flowers form elongated conical spikes at the tops of the stems.

FLAVOR

Strong hot menthol taste and fragrance from the volatile oil which is present in all aerial parts.

PARTS USED

Leaves and flowers.

HOW TO GROW

Type: invasive, hardy perennial, native to Europe and Asia
Exposure: part shade; moist, well-drained soil
Propagation: from root cuttings
Harvesting: clip back during growing season and especially when flowering

HEALING PROPERTIES

Actions: antispasmodic, digestive tonic, prevents vomiting, carminative, peripheral vasodilator, promotes sweating, promotes bile flow, analgesic

Uses: Peppermint's main benefit lies in its mild anesthetic effect on the mucous membranes, which helps quell nausea and vomiting.
Taking peppermint, preferably before eating, helps stimulate liver and gall bladder function by

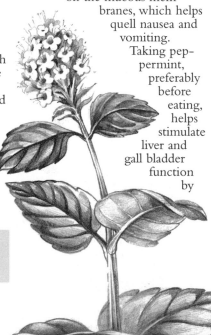

increasing bile flow to the liver and intestines. This extra bile helps break down fats and allows the body to more efficiently use the fats. It also acts as an intestinal and stomach disinfectant, preventing fermentation of undigested food, thus helping stop gas production. It is used in ulcerative colitis, Crohn's Disease, diverticular disease, travel sickness, fevers, colds, flu, and to improve the appetite.

Phytochemistry: Menthol is the constituent that gives peppermint its antiseptic, decongestant, analgelistic and mildly anesthetic (the cooling, numbing sensation) properties.

CAUTION

Never apply peppermint oil to the noses of infants or small children (or give them peppermint tea); the menthol vapors can cause choking. It is contraindicated in pregnancy due to the strongly stimulating oil.

AVAILABILITY

Fresh sprigs in some markets and supermarkets. Dried leaves in alternative/health stores. Teas widely available.

HOW TO USE IN COOKING

Whole sprigs: in sauces; as a garnish; in teas or drinks.
Leaves: fresh or dried in jellies, sauces, teas, beverages, desserts, salads, marinades, vegetable and fruit dishes.
Flowers: fresh, chopped into salads, stir-fries, vegetable and fruit dishes.
Peppermint tea from fresh or dried leaves and flowers is delicious hot or iced. Blend peppermint with other tea herbs to lend flavor.

FOLKLORE

The Ancients used mint to scent their bath water and as a restorative. The Athenians perfumed each part of their body with a different scent, mint being used for the arms. As early as 1704, Ray's *Historia Plantarum* was claiming "peper mint" to be a superior mint for treating "stomach weakness" and diarrhea. By 1721, peppermint leaves had attained official status in the *London Pharmacopoeia*.

Rosemary
Rosmarinus officinalis

DESCRIPTION

An evergreen shrub that grows to 6 feet (180 cm) in warmer climates. Needle-like, leathery leaves are about 1 inch (2.5 cm) long, linear and dark green. Pale blue flowers grow in clusters towards the ends of the branches. New shoots are downy and later become woody with greyish-brown, scaly bark.

FLAVOR

Camphorous; a blend of ginger, mint, lemon and pine.

PARTS USED

Flowers and leaves.

HOW TO GROW

Type: tender perennial, hardy to zone 6, native to the Mediterranean
Exposure: full sun; dry, well-drained, chalky soil, sheltered; protect from frost
Propagation: seeds, cuttings and division of roots
Harvesting: clip sprigs all season

HEALING PROPERTIES

Actions: antioxidant, anti-cancer, anti-inflammatory, astringent, nervine, carminative, antiseptic, diuretic, diaphoretic, promotes bile flow, antidepressant, circulatory stimulant, antispasmodic, nervous system and cardiac tonic

Uses: Researchers at the Nestle Research Centre in Switzerland recently found that whole rosemary extracts prevented DNA damage in cell cultures induced by aflatoxin, a potent agent known to cause liver cancer. Animal studies give strong evidence that rosemary may be effective in preventing breast cancer in humans. Rosemary contains anti-inflammatory chemical components that fight against the deterioration of brain functions — which shows some degree of truth to its ancient symbolism as the herb for remembrance. As a circulatory stimulant and antispasmodic, it is useful in migraine headache. As a circulatory stimulant it is used in chronic fatigue syndrome, to improve memory — and for hair loss, since it improves the blood circulation to the head. Rosemary's effectiveness as a food preservative equals that of the synthetic food preservatives butylated hydroxyanisole (BHA) and butylated hydroxytoluene (BHT).

Phytochemistry: Two antioxidants in rosemary — carnosol and carnosic acid — are believed to be the cancer-fighting agents. Carvacrol and other compounds found in rosemary protect acetylcholine, a chemical messenger in the brain, the loss of which is linked to Alzheimer's disease.

Food value (dried, per 100 g): 1280 mg calcium; 70 mg phosphorus; 29 mg iron; 3,128 I.U. beta carotene; 61 mg vitamin C.

CAUTION

Avoid large amounts during pregnancy as uterine contractions may occur.

AVAILABILITY

Whole, fresh sprigs found in some ethnic markets and supermarkets. Dried whole and powdered leaf found in supermarkets, health/alternative stores.

How to use in cooking

Sprig: fresh flowering sprigs to flavor vinegar, oils and wine; fresh woody sprigs as a skewer for grilling meats and vegetables, tied together as a brush to add sauce to foods on the grill; dried in *bouquet garnis* and to release flavor when burned with coals for grilling foods

Leaf: whole in soups, stocks and long-simmering dishes; chopped fresh or dried with fruit (melons or citrus), wine punch, lamb, poultry, marinades, stuffings, stews; teams nicely with garlic for roasted vegetable dishes; ground fresh or dried to season mashed potatoes, puddings, sauces and baked goods such as breads, scones, brownies and pastry.

For picnics or outdoor events, sprinkle a generous helping of crushed rosemary leaves into potato or pasta salad for flavor and to keep food from spoiling.

Folklore

The name translates from the Latin *ros marinus* to "dew of the sea." Rosemary is the symbol for remembrance and as such, it holds a special position among herbs, being used at weddings (entwined in the bridal wreath and gilded for gifts), at New Year's, at funerals, at festivals, as incense in religious ceremonies, by students, to show friendship, and in magical spells. From *Banckes' Herbal*: "Smell it oft and it shall keep thee youngly."

Sage
Salvia officinalis

Description

A hardy, low-growing shrub (to 1 foot [30 cm]). Soft, long, oval, greyish green leaves grow on downy herbaceous stems at the top of a woody base. Pink, purple, blue or white tubular flowers grow in whorls at the top of stems.

How to grow

Type: hardy perennial, native to northern Mediterranean coast
Exposure: full sun; dry, well-drained soil
Propagation: seeds or cuttings
Harvesting: clip sprigs all season

Flavor

Pungent, camphorous, lemony.

Healing properties

Actions: antioxidant, antimicrobial, antibiotic, antiseptic, carminative, antispasmodic, anti-inflammatory, estrogenic, peripheral vasodilator, reduces perspiration, uterine stimulant

Uses: Sage's volatile oil kills bacteria and fungi, even those resistant to penicillin. Sage also dries up phlegm and is especially useful as a gargle in sore throat, laryngitis and mouth ulcers. Singers with laryngitis have used it for relief and gone on to perform the same day. It is used to relieve night sweats and hot flashes of menopause.

Food value (dried, per 100 g): 1,652 mg calcium; 91 mg phosphorus; 28 mg iron; 11 mg niacin, 1,070 mg potassium; 5,900 I.U. beta carotene; 5.7 mg niacin; 32 mg vitamin C.

Caution

Sage can cause convulsions in very high doses. If taking large doses of sage tea (3 or more cups per day), do not use for longer than 1 week. Do not use where high blood pressure or epilepsy is evident. Do not use sage in medicinal doses during pregnancy as it can cause contractions of the uterus.

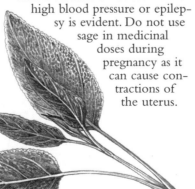

Availability

Fresh sprigs at some supermarkets and farmers' markets; dried, whole, cut, rubbed or ground at supermarkets

Parts used

Leaves and flowers.

How to use in cooking

Sage is the main ingredient in poultry seasoning, thus it goes best with poultry and fowl.
Sprig: fresh, in soups, stews and long-simmering sauces, as a stuffing with onions for whole fish to be baked; fresh flowering sprigs to flavor vinegar, oils and wine; as a garnish dried to release flavor when burned with coals for grilling foods
Leaf: fresh or dried with lamb, pork; use in cheese dishes, stuffings, dressings and tomato sauces, marinades, breads. For a throat-soothing tea, blend sage with sweet cicely, mint and/or licorice.
Flower: chopped fresh in salads, vegetable dishes; as a garnish.

Folklore

Cur moriatur homo cui Salvia crescit in horto? — Why should a man die while sage grows in his garden? This Latin saying gives an indication of the high regard the Ancients held for the medicinal properties of this plant.
From *The Cook's Oracle*, 1821: "Sage and Onion Sauce" "Chop very fine an ounce of onion and 1/2 oz. of green Sage leaves, put them in a stamper with 4 spoonsful of water, simmer gently for 10 minutes, then put in a teaspoonful of pepper and salt and 1 oz. of fine breadcrumbs. Mix well together, then pour to it 1/2 pint of Broth, Gravy or Melted Butter, stir well together and simmer a few minutes longer. This is a relishing sauce for Roast Pork, Geese or Duck, or with Green Peas on Maigre Days."

Sea Herbs

Marine algae, the edible, wild plants of the oceans (often called seaweeds or sea vegetables), of which there are many different kinds, have been harvested by seaside communities around the world and cultures of the Far East for centuries. They are primitive plants with blades for leaves, stipes for stems and holdfasts for roots. The high concentration of minerals and their abundant vitamins (exceptionally high amounts of vitamin A), along with carbohydrates and a small amount of protein, make them valuable additions to a healthy diet. Most sea herbs have anti-cancer properties.

Arame *Eisenia bicyclis*
Primary source: Japan's northern and southern coasts
Appearance: dark yellow-brown when growing, black when dried, short, thin, curled strands
Taste and texture: soft, slightly resistant texture, sweet, delicate flavor
Healing properties: alleviates high blood pressure, builds strong bones and teeth; one of the richest source of iodine, highly concentrated in iron and calcium
Preparation: soak in water 3 to 5 minutes, then cook as directed in recipe, or add to long-simmering soups and stews directly.
How to use in cooking: in curries salads, soups, stews, tomato sauce

Dulse *Palmaria palmata*
Primary source: North Atlantic waters
Appearance: large, dark red fronds
Taste and texture: chewy, nutlike, salt taste
Healing properties: cooling, prevents scurvy, induces sweating, remedy for seasickness and the herpes virus; exceptionally concentrated in iodine, which is important to the thyroid gland; rich in manganese, which activates the enzyme system. Dulse is a good source of phosphorus, B vitamins, vitamins E and

C, bromine, potassium, magnesium, sulfur, calcium, sodium, radium, boron, rubidium, manganese, titanium, and other trace elements.
Preparation: soak in water 20 minutes, then cook as directed in recipe, or add to long-simmering soups and stews directly.
How to use in cooking: use whole the same way as spinach; chopped, in stuffings, relishes, salad dressings; toast and eat as a snack; thickens gravies and sauces

Hijiki *Hizikia fusiforme*
Primary source: Japan's northern and southern coasts
Appearance: brown when fresh, black when dried; short, thin, curled strands
Taste and texture: sweet, delicate flavor; crisp
Healing properties: diuretic, resolves heat-induced phlegm, detoxifies the body, benefits thyroid, moistens hardness, helps normalize blood sugar levels, aids weight loss, soothes nerves, supports hormone functions, builds bones and teeth; an excellent source of calcium, iron and iodine, and abundant in vitamin B2 and niacin.
Preparation: soak in water 15 to 20 minutes, then cook as directed in recipe, or add to long-simmering soups and stews directly.
How to use in cooking: in salads and rice dishes, soups, stews, stuffings, stir-fries

Nori *Porphyra tenera*
Primary source: both coasts of North America, middle and lower tidal zones of sea coasts, called "laver" in Britain
Appearance: bright pink when young, dark purple when older; leaves pressed into thin sheets
Taste and texture: like mild, salty corn; toasted sheets

Healing properties: antibacterial, diuretic, treats painful urination, goiter, edema, high blood pressure, beriberi, appears to heal ulcers; is high in protein and rich in vitamins A, C, B1, niacin and phosphorus
Preparation: toast sheets lightly over a low flame or element on high until black and crisp.
How to use in cooking (sheets): wrap vegetables and rice for sushi; *(chopped or crumbled):* add to salads, stir-fries, vegetable dishes.

Wakame *Undaria pinnatifida*
Primary source: Japan's northern seas
Appearance: thin, black fronds
Taste and texture: softly resistant texture; strong, sweet flavor.
Healing properties: boosts immune functioning, promotes healthy hair and skin; used in Japanese tradition to purify mother's blood after childbirth; rich in calcium, niacin and thiamin.
Preparation: soak in water 5 minutes, drain and simmer 45 minutes.
How to use in cooking (whole): as any leafy green vegetable, in soups, stews, salads, sandwiches, vegetable and stir-fry dishes; *(chopped):* in spreads and with whole grains.

Kelp *Pleurophycus gardneri*
Primary source: Pacific coast of North America
Appearance: broad, leaf-like fronds, light brown to light olive-brown
Taste and texture: usually available in granular, powdered or tablet form; fresh or dried frond has a delicate, mild taste when cooked
Healing properties: antibacterial, antiviral (herpes), may lower blood pressure and cholesterol; high in calcium, phosphorus, and iodine
Preparation: none, if granular or powdered; rehydrate if dried
How to use in cooking (fresh): wrap around rice or other fillings; *(steamed or baked):* chop and added to stir-fries, salads or stuffings; *(powdered):* sprinkle into soups, stews, salads, stir-fries; mix with dry ingredients in breads, muffins; *(granular):* add to most dishes, sauces, gravy, dips and spreads; *(powder):* mix with other salt substitute herbs.

Dulse

Kelp

Thyme
Thymus

DESCRIPTION
A bushy, low-growing shrub with several many-branched stems. Opposite, small, oblong leaves grow right out of the stems that are woody almost to the tip. Pink, purple or white tubular flowers grow in terminal clusters, covering the plant.

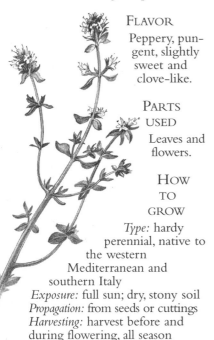

FLAVOR
Peppery, pungent, slightly sweet and clove-like.

PARTS USED
Leaves and flowers.

HOW TO GROW
Type: hardy perennial, native to the western Mediterranean and southern Italy
Exposure: full sun; dry, stony soil
Propagation: from seeds or cuttings
Harvesting: harvest before and during flowering, all season

HEALING PROPERTIES
Actions: antioxidant, expectorant, antiseptic, antispasmodic, astringent, tonic, antimicrobial, antibiotic, heals wounds, diuretic, soothes coughs, nervine

Uses: Thyme is ideal for deep-seated chest infections such as chronic coughs and bronchitis. For throat infections, it can be used as a gargle.
Phytochemistry: Scottish researchers found that among the 75 chemicals found in in thyme extract, 25% of them had antioxidant properties.
Thymol and carvacrol are the active ingredients that make thyme act as an expectorant.

Food value: 1,890 mg calcium; 201 mg phosphorus; 123 mg iron; 814 mg potassium; 3,800 I.U. beta carotene; 4.9 mg niacin

CAUTION
Avoid in pregnancy. Children under 2 years of age and people with thyroid problems should not be given/take medicinal preparations of thyme.

AVAILABILITY
Fresh sprigs in some markets; dried whole leaves in alternative/health stores.

HOW TO USE IN COOKING
Thyme is extremely versatile and can be added to most dishes; it stands up to long cooking in soups, stews, tomato sauces, gumbos, chowders. Used daily, its antioxidant effect will be beneficial. Use thyme in canning and preserving because of its antibacterial, anti-fungal activity.
Sprig: fresh flowering sprigs in fruit and vegetable preserves, to flavor vinegar, oils and wine, in long-simmering dishes; dried in *bouquet garnis* and to release flavor when burned with coals for grilling foods
Leaf: fresh in salads; fresh or dried with meats, vegetable dishes, soups, casseroles, stuffings, pâtés, sausages, breads, mayonnaise, vinegars, mustards, in herb blends. Use lemon thyme with seafood and fish dishes; lemon-flavored baked goods and desserts
Flower: fresh, in vinegars, butters and sauces; as a garnish on soups, pasta, rice and desserts. Dried leaves and flowers are blended with other tea herbs.

FOLKLORE
The emperor Charlemagne ordered thyme grown in all of his gardens because he valued its medicinal and culinary properties. The Greeks knew of and used thyme's antiseptic properties — it was burned to cleanse and perfume the air and to repel insects.

Turmeric
Curcuma longa

DESCRIPTION
A deciduous perennial belonging to the *zingiberaceate* (ginger) family, turmeric is a long rhizome resembling ginger but thinner and rounder. The flesh is brilliant orange with a covering of thin, brownish skin. Growing rhizomes sprout 2- to 4-foot (60 to 120 cm) shoots with broad, glossy, lance-shaped leaves.

FLAVOR
Flavor is at its peak in freshly grated turmeric, which is pungent and charged with a fresh, peppery, camphorous, slightly acrid taste. Dried, whole rhizomes retain a warm, sweetish, woody character. Dried, powdered turmeric is weaker and slightly bitter in taste but still gives a yellow color to foods.

PARTS USED
Rhizome.

HOW TO GROW
Type: Tender perennial, hardy to zone 10, native to Southeast Asia,
Exposure: Full sun; moist soil; outside in the sun

LEFT: SWEET POTATO CRISPS WITH LAVENDER AÏOLI (PAGE 54) ➤
RIGHT: VEGETABLE SUSHI WITH WASABI MAYONNAISE DIP (PAGE 62)

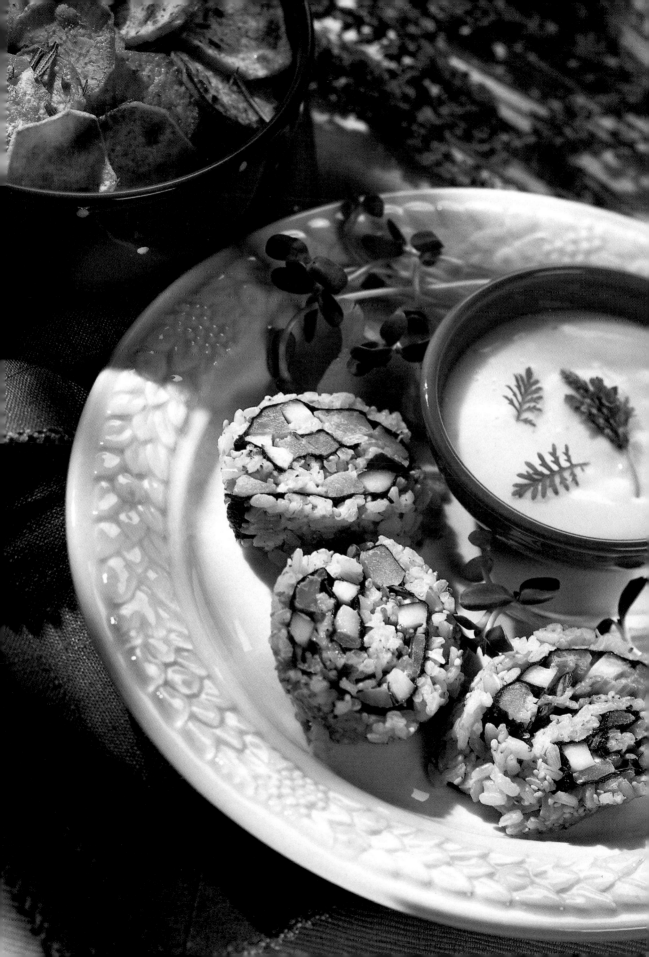

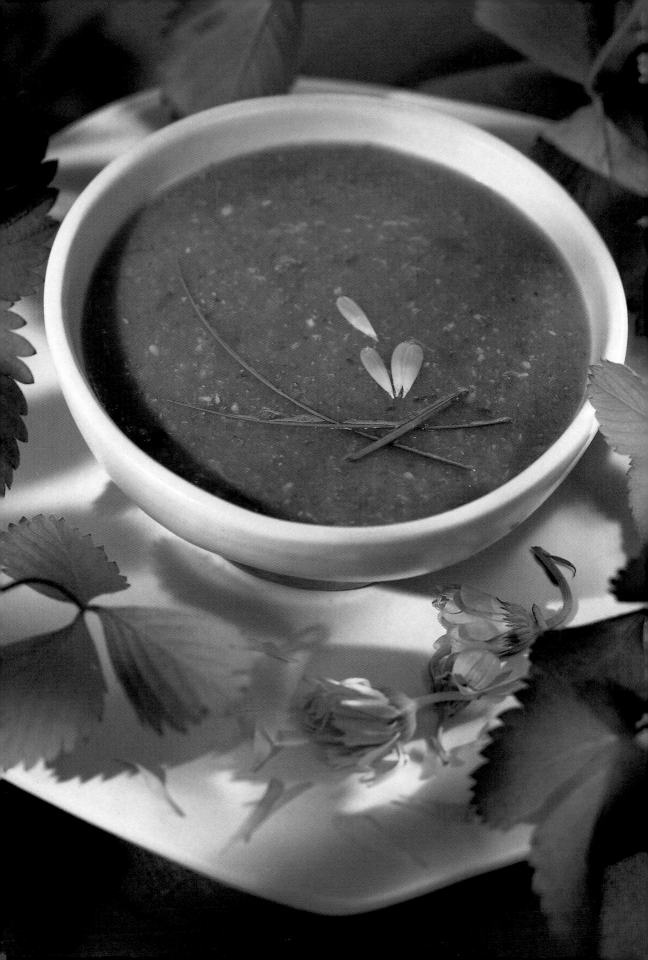

belt, summer outdoors and winter indoors in colder regions
Propagation: By replanting fingers broken from the mother plant

HEALING PROPERTIES

Actions: antioxidant, anti-inflammatory, antimicrobial (against *staphylococcus aureus*), antibacterial, anti-fungal, antiviral, anticoagulant, analgesic, anti-cancer, hinders the buildup of cholesterol plaques in arteries, reduces post-exercise pain, heals wounds, antispasmodic, reduction of intestinal gas formation, protects liver cells, increases bile production and bile flow, potential antitumor activity

Uses: Curcumin in turmeric is as effective as the preservative BHA and appears to inhibit the development of colon cancer, according to animal studies carried out by the American Health Foundation in Valhalla, N.Y. Curcumin has also been shown to inhibit breast tumors in rats. Turmeric is used in eczema, liver disease (such as hepatitis), nausea, digestive disturbances, debility due to recent illness or operation; in cooking, it aids fat and protein digestion, especially where the gall bladder has been removed. In diabetes it boosts insulin activity; its anticoagulant action helps protect the heart and blood vessels and reduces the risk of stroke in people with heart problems or a history of previous strokes. Its circulatory stimulant, antioxidant and anti-inflammatory actions are useful in rheumatoid arthritis and gout.

Phytochemistry: A group of chemicals known as curcuminoids is considered the most important contributor to the herb's activity. The best known of the curcuminoids is curcumin, the bright yellow pigment in turmeric. Borneol oil is anti-inflammatory and valepotriates (constituents of the relaxing herb valerian) are responsible for its analgesic action.

AVAILABILITY

Asian stores stock fresh or frozen whole rhizomes, Oriental markets or natural food stores offer the dried, whole rhizomes, and supermarkets sell ground turmeric.

HOW TO USE IN COOKING

Turmeric is one of the ingredients in traditional Indian curries. Use the fresh root whenever possible, cutting or grating it as required. If using slices or julienned strips, remove from the dish before serving. Use turmeric to add a warm, clean, camphorous note and a bright yellow hue to rice dishes, cheeses, lentils, pickles, chicken, fish, salsas and liqueurs. Blend with other spices/herbs: sweet (cinnamon or cloves); hot (pepper or mustard); earthy (cumin or fenugreek); sharp (dill, bay or thyme).
Fresh: whole in stocks, soups, stews; sliced to flavor vinegars, oils soups or stocks; julienned in stir-fries; finely chopped or grated, raw in salad dressings, marinades; cooked in all main dishes, stir-fries, preserves and pickles; juice to flavor salad dressings, marinades or sauces; candied in fruit salads, salad dressings and sauces.
To store fresh root: in a cool, dry place for several days; wrap in a paper towel and set in an open plastic bag to keep for several weeks in the refrigerator; seal fresh root in plastic bag, freeze and cut off as needed or peel and slice, place in a glass jar, cover with vodka, seal and refrigerate (keeps indefinitely); candied turmeric keeps for a year or longer, and is easy to use in cooking. (See page 40 for information on preparing candied roots.)
Dried: ground, in cooking as you would fresh.
Leaves: as a decorative plate liner, to wrap fish for the grill, or to serve finger foods.

FOLKLORE

Turmeric is mentioned in India's ancient Ayurveda, suggesting that is has been used for over 3,000 years. Ancient Persians associated it and other yellow spices with sun worship. The Chinese have used it in traditional medicine since the 7th century. Indians used it to treat leprosy and jaundice and they still consume large amounts of it — a practice encouraged by the Indian government for its health benefits. Perhaps for the same reason, the U.S. armed forces had a strict guideline regarding the composition of curry used in military mess halls: Federal Military Specification EE-S-631 stipulated that 37 to 39 percent of the spices had to be turmeric.

Other Edible Healing Herbs

Ginkgo *Ginkgo biloba*

Actions: anti-oxidant, memory enhancer, relaxes blood vessels, circulatory stimulant
Uses: Ginkgo increases blood flow to the brain and it also produces a significant rise in dopamine synthesis, a neurotransmitter that is critical to the transfer of information and electrochemical impulses between nerves and other nerves, and between nerves and muscles, glands, organs, blood vessels and other structures of the body. These functions are what allow ginkgo leaf extract to improve short-term memory, increase concentration, quicken information recall, and enhance alertness. Ginkgo is very useful in the treatment and prevention of premature aging and studies have shown that ginkgo can help stabilize or even improve the memory of people with Alzheimer's disease.
How to use in cooking: In most studies of

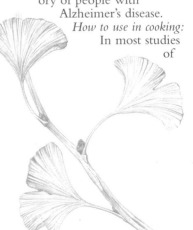

ginkgo, subjects have taken 120 to 240 mg a day of standardized leaf extracts for from 4 weeks to 9 months; you can't expect the same results with fresh or dried leaves, since they dol not provide the same quantity of active components. The amounts used in cooking will not have a significant effect on the body. However, using dried ginkgo leaves in stocks, soups and teas is recommended if they are readily available.

Raspberry *Rubus idaeus*

Actions - Leaves: astringent, preparative for childbirth, stimulant, digestive remedy, tonic; *Fruit:* diuretic, laxative, diaphoretic, cleansing; a good source of vitamins and minerals

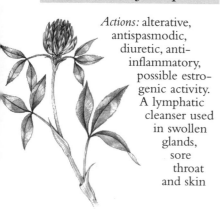

How to use in cooking (leaves): whole or crushed in soups, stock, tea blends; *(berries):* whole in salads, desserts; crushed in syrups, vinegars, sauces, desserts; juice in syrups, sauces, beverages

Red Clover *Trifolium pratense*

Actions: alterative, antispasmodic, diuretic, anti-inflammatory, possible estrogenic activity. A lymphatic cleanser used in swollen glands, sore throat and skin

disease. During the 1930s, red clover was prescribed as an anticancer remedy.
How to use in cooking (whole flowers): in tea blends, soups, stock, as a garnish; *(petals):* red petals removed from green center: fresh or dried, in sauces, dressings, stuffing; dessert sauces and puddings

Rose *Rosa*

Actions: antidepressant, antispasmodic, astringent, sedative, digestive, stimulant, increases bile production, cleansing, expectorant, antibacterial, antiviral, antiseptic, kidney tonic, blood tonic menstrual regulator, anti-inflammatory
How to use in cooking - Petals: use to flavor syrups and sauces; *Hips:* an important source of vitamin C, use fresh or dried rosehips in teas, syrups and fruit drinks, steep in water, then add to stocks, soups, sauces and gravy; *Water:* used in desserts and dessert sauces

St. John's Wort
Hypericum perforatum

Actions: antidepressant, astringent, analgesic, anti-inflammatory, sedative, restorative tonic for the nervous system
How to use in cooking -Flowering tops: fresh or dried, in stocks, soups, stews; *Flowers and Petals:* in stocks, soups, salads, sauces, as a garnish, in teas and tea blends

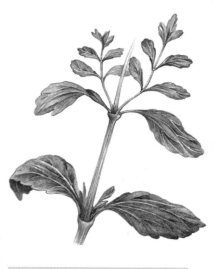

Stevia *Stevia rebaudiana*

Actions: energy booster; natural sweetener without calories, tonic, digestive, diuretic
How to use in cooking: One teaspoon (5 mL) of dried stevia leaves is sweeter than 1 cup (250 mL) sugar.
Whole sprigs: make a tea from a handful of fresh sprigs and 2 cups (500 mL) boiling water, let steep overnight; strain, then add liquid to sauces, dressings, puddings and other desserts.
Leaves: fresh or dried, make a tea and use as a sweetener as listed above.
Powder: substitute 2 tbsp (25 mL) stevia powder for 1 cup (250 mL) sugar in recipes.
Liquid: add drops to tea, juices and other beverages to sweeten.
Note: Some sugar is required for the success of baked goods, so stevia cannot be substituted for sugar in all recipes.

COOKING WITH MEDICINAL HERBS

*Herbs are the friends of physicians
and the praise of cooks.*
Emperor Charlemagne

THE MEDICINAL EFFECT OF HERBS IN COOKING

There are several traditional ways of using medicinal plants. For thousands of years, ordinary folk have treated everyday problems with simple herbal remedies in the form of salves, teas and poultices. Monks and, after them, herbalists still employ tinctures and standardized doses in capsules or pre-measured doses. Chinese, Ayurvedic and homeopathic medicines evolved highly organized systems of natural healing using plants. I would like to propose that there is one other, richly rewarding way of using these same medicinal plants, and that is to cook with them.

Not that the notion of cooking with healing herbs is new to humans. Over many centuries, Chinese cooks have developed a time-honored cuisine that relies on a multitude of barks, roots, seeds and herbs, cherished for their restorative powers. And we in Canada and the United States don't have to go far back in our nations' history to find a people for whom their food was their medicine. Technical study confirms the physical endurance of North American Indians before European explorers (pre-1492) and reveals none of our modern-day bone deficiency, cavities, arthritis, tuberculosis, cancer, polio and other "modern" diseases in these peoples. In fact, the natural diet of the North American Indian — which included indigenous herbs, plants, berries, nuts, seeds, fish, fowl and game — was incredibly health-supporting.

On the other hand, our diet of refined, processed, fat- and chemical-laden foods is killing us. And the fastest way back to that health-supporting relationship with food is to follow a "lean green" diet. In addition, the journey back to a natural diet should be via the herb garden. People everywhere — urban apartment dwellers included — can grow and have access to fresh organic herbs seasonally and a dried supply in winter. Growing herbs allows us to understand the properties of each plant as we read about and experiment first-hand with teas and other simple remedies and make them a part of our daily meals.

The use of herbs for specific therapeutic results is affected by a number of environmental and lifestyle factors, including (but not limited to) what we eat. Herbalists employ herbs of which they know the strength of the active ingredients and the method of preparing and administering the doses. Cooking with medicinal herbs does not yield the same reliable treatment. However, if we consistently cook with fresh, whole, organic ingredients and include a variety of herbs in everyday meals, we will enjoy a preventative effect from this healthy style of eating. By healthy eating choices, we can increase resistance to modern diseases, build our immune system and strengthen the functioning of organs and other bodily systems.

Healing and good health is possible for all. It always requires a commitment and dedication as well as a willingness to change — to give up one way of thinking and acting in order to embrace a new way of being. In addition, most genuine healing requires a cleansing process (including purifying emotions, home and work environments, and internal body cleansing); a diet change and the addition of specific doses of herbs or plant compounds; daily aerobic exercise; stress reduction; increasing emotional support resources; and an attempt to deepen our connection to the creative force (whatever that may be for each of us). All of these issues are connected to lifestyle and whether we like it or not, the choices we make either nourish or destroy us.

Health is wholeness and balance. Many herbalists believe that using nutrition as a preventative tool for promoting health is one-third of the total picture — exercise and spiritual nurturing being the other parts of the equation. As aboriginal societies proved, when these three combine to support inner resilience, you can experience the inevitable interactions with germs and not get infections; you can be in contact with allergens and not suffer allergies; and you can be exposed to carcinogens and not get cancer.

PRESERVING HERBS FOR COOKING OR MEDICINAL USE

Traditional methods of preserving herbs and foods were: drying; salting; and keeping in vinegar, sugar, fat or alcohol. The cook and herbalist had no other means of saving the fresh harvest for use during winter. Drying was the most popular method of ensuring a steady supply of herbs at times when they were not available fresh. However, herbalists have used and continue to use tinctures (active components of herbs condensed and preserved in alcohol), simple salves (active components of herbs preserved in lard, grease or oil) and herbal syrups and honeys to assist in the practice of using herbs for health. We can borrow from the culinary tradition of preserving whole herbs in vinegars and oils by using the same techniques for medicinal herbs.

How To Dry Herbs

Most herbs dry well, the exceptions being parsley, chives and basil, which are better frozen. To dry well, herbs require a warm, dry, dark atmosphere where air circulates freely — a closet, attic, dark corner of a room, basement or a barn.

To Dry Bunches: For long-stemmed herbs (mints, yarrow, sage), gather in small bunches, tie stems and hang upside down in a warm, dry, dark place. Some people use paper bags to catch the falling bits and to keep the light away.

To Dry Leaves or Petals: For leaves on short stems (violets, coltsfoot) and flowers (calendula, violets, and all others), strip leaves off the stems and petals off the center of the flower, or dry the flowerhead whole. Scatter leaves or petals in a single layer on a nylon net or screen. The faster the plant parts dry, the more color and fragrance they will retain.

To Dry Roots: Scrub, cut into 1/2-inch (1 cm) pieces, and place in one layer on a drying rack, screen or suspended fabric to dry. Leave in pieces for longer storage. Grind small amounts to a powder just before using. Bottle and store in dark-colored bottles in a cool, dark place.

To Store Dried Herbs: Use dark-colored glass or ceramic containers with tight-fitting lids to store herbs individually. Label and date and keep in a cool, dark place for no longer than 1 year.

Medicinal Teas

Second only to water as a world beverage, tea has been cultivated and harvested since at least the 4th century.. The medicinal benefits of herbal teas have long been part of Asian tradition and now, through increasing scientific study, Westerners are learning that certain teas aid digestion, are antibacterial, contain antioxidants (to help the body resist aging), and help prevent cancer, along with many other health-promoting properties. Teas are effective as a therapeutic tool because when boiling water is

poured over a herb and the herb is allow to steep, the herb's cell walls are broken, releasing its soluble organic compounds and essences into the water (and steam).

While fresh herbs can be used to make nutritive teas, most medicinal tea recipes call for (and the amounts are specific to) dried herbs because dried herbs are easiest to store, transport and use. In the recipes for herbal teas (pages 37-38), amounts given are for dried herbs. When substituting fresh herbs for dried in any recipe, use the following formula: *1 tbsp (15 mL) fresh herbs = 1 tsp (5 mL) dried herbs.*

Just as commercial tea producers blend several tea leaves for each kind of tea, so herbalists have learned that combining different herb leaves, flowers, roots and seeds, or adding certain others will boost a tea's potency. When a specific medicinal benefit is desired from a tea, blending stevia, sweet cicely, or licorice for sweetness and flavor, and lemon balm, mint, or basil for extra taste, will not take away from the herb's healing quality. Licorice is an excellent herb to add to herb blends because of its ability to enhance the medicinal effect of other herbs.

Drying and Blending Herbs for Teas

Follow instructions above for drying herbs. Strip leaves from the stems, but try to keep the leaves whole for long-term storage; crushing or grinding them releases the essential oils and the medicinal components. Blend the dried whole leaves, petals, seeds and chopped dried roots according to your needs or the suggested combinations below. Store in a labeled airtight tin or dark-colored jar in a dark, cool place. When ready to use in teas, grind enough for 2 to 3 days (about 1/2 cup [125 mL]) to a fine powder; store in a dark jar.

Tea Terms

Decoction: A solution obtained by using the woody parts of plants (roots, seeds, bark) and boiling them in water 10 to 20 minutes.

Tea: Strictly speaking, "tea" refers to a solution made by pouring boiling water on the fermented leaves and stems of a plant which have been allowed to dry after fermentation (green or black tea). The term is often used when referring to a solution made by pouring boiling water on any plant's leaves, petals or stems.

Tisane: The correct term used for steeping fresh or dried herbs in boiling water. Interchangeable with "tea" when herbs are used.

How to Brew Healing Tea

Herb teas should be made and used immediately as the volatile oils evaporate and the taste and medicinal benefit can be dispersed in the steam. Bring fresh cold filtered water to the boil. Rinse a teapot with some of the boiling water, and pour off. Do not use metal teapots and keep a teapot strictly for medicinal teas. Measure 1 tbsp (15 mL) crushed herbs per 1 cup (250 mL) into the warmed pot. If making more than 2 cups of tea, add an extra tablespoon (15 mL) dried herbs "for the pot." Pour boiling filtered water over, put a lid on the pot and a stopper in the spout, let steep 5 to 10 minutes and strain into cups.

How to Brew Healing Decoctions

Follow directions on page 36 for drying roots. Crush, then grind roots, seeds and bark in a mortar or food processor or coffee grinder. Measure 1 tbsp (15 mL) roots per 1 cup (250 mL) into a non-reactive pot. Cover with filtered water and lid. Bring to a boil and adjust heat to keep mixture simmering for 10 to 20 minutes. Allow to cool slightly in pot; strain into cups.

Medicinal Benefits of Teas

In order to feel specific healing effects of herbs through teas, it is usually recommended that a decoction or tisane be taken three to five times per day for a period of one month for every year you have suffered from the ailment. What follows are suggestions for some healing teas.

DIGESTIVE TEA

Allspice (*Pimenta dioica*) is a pungent, warming herb, the dried berries being most commonly available although leaves are also used medicinally.

Actions: improves digestion, tonic for nervous system, antiseptic, anesthetic

1 cup	dried peppermint leaves	250 mL
1/2 cup	chopped, dried dandelion roots	125 mL
1/4 cup	whole allspice berries	50 mL
2 tbsp	ground ginger	25 mL
1	1-inch (2.5 cm) piece licorice root, crushed	1

1. Blend ingredients together, store in an airtight jar in a dark, cool place.

To make one cup of tea: pour 1 cup (250 mL) boiling water over 1 tbsp (15 mL) tea blend. Drink hot with a meal.
Makes: 2 cups (500 mL), about 30 cups of tea.

Substitute: 2 tbsp (25 mL) ground for whole allspice berries; 2 tbsp (25 mL) ground for licorice root
Benefits: Soothes and comforts the stomach, intestines, nerves and glands, including the pancreas and liver.

STRESS-REDUCING TEA

Linden (*Tilia x europaea*), native to Europe but grown in Canada and the United States, is also known as Limeflower or Tilia.

1 cup	lemon balm leaves	250 mL
1 cup	linden leaves	250 mL
1/4 cup	valerian root, crushed	50 mL
1 tbsp	crushed ginger root	15 mL

1. Blend ingredients together, store in an airtight jar in a dark, cool place.

To make one cup of tea: pour 1 cup (250 mL) boiling water over 1 tbsp (15 mL) tea blend. Drink while still hot before retiring or just before a time of quiet. For best results, sip the tea while relaxing in a warm bath to which a few drops of essential oil of jasmine, lavender or rose has been added.
Makes: 2 1/4 cups (550 mL), about 35 cups of tea.
Substitute: Chamomile flowers for linden leaves
Benefits: Soothes nerves, relaxes and acts as a mild sedative.

PAIN- AND INFLAMMATION-REDUCING TEA

For best results, sip the tea while relaxing in a warm bath to which a few drops of essential oil of St. John's wort has been added.

1 cup	alfalfa leaves and flowers	250 mL
1 cup	chamomile leaves	250 mL
1/4 cup	dried ginger root, crushed	50 mL
3 tbsp	crushed willow bark	45 mL
1 tbsp	crushed ginger root	15 mL

1. Blend ingredients together, store in an airtight jar in a dark, cool place.

To make one cup of tea: Pour 1 cup (250 mL) boiling water over 1 tbsp (15 mL) tea blend. Drink while still hot before retiring or just before a time of quiet.
Makes: 2 1/4 cups (550 mL), about 35 cups of tea.
Omit: Willow bark if not available
Benefits: Reduces swelling, helps to reduce pain of arthritis.

HEALING HERBAL TEAS

Problem	Healing Herbal Tea
acne	lemon balm, stinging nettle
anxiety	chamomile, St. John's wort, lemon balm
canker sores	calendula, sage
colic (in babies)	fennel seeds, sage
constipation	burdock root, licorice
coughs	coltsfoot, hyssop, horehound, borage, elder, garlic, licorice
common cold symptoms	echinacea, astragalus, chamomile
infection	garlic, cinnamon, cloves
mild depression	St. John's wort, basil
fever	hyssop, echinacea
gastritis	calendula
high blood pressure	garlic, green tea
menstrual pain, problems	calendula, chamomile, motherwort
nausea, indigestion	ginger, chamomile, basil
sore throat, tonsillitis	sage, thyme

JUICES

Raw herb, vegetable and fruit juices have a higher concentration of nutrients than the whole. While some elements are lost or become insoluble during drying and heating (cooking), fresh plant juice captures the whole synergistic complex of healing ingredients within the living cells of the plant. Use organic produce and just scrub, do not peel. Juice small amounts at a time and keep extra in refrigerator no longer than 1 day. Use plant juices in soup stocks, sauces, marinades and salad dressings or wherever "stock" is called for in recipes.

To Extract Juice from Roots

The goodness from fresh roots such as ginger, ginseng, burdock and dandelion can be obtained without a juice extractor. To do this, cut the root into large chunks (if organic, leave skin on) and spin in the food processor or blender for a minute or two, until the particles are quite small. If you don't have access to a food processor or blender, grate or cut and smash the roots with a knife until they become pulpy. Place the pulp in a square of muslin or cheesecloth and wring out the juice into a cup.

To Use Herb Juices in Cooking

Do not strain off the starchy residue that settles to the bottom of squeezed juice — stir it into the juice before using. One pound (500 g) of fresh root yields approximately 1/3 cup (75 mL) juice. Use 2 tbsp (25 mL) of herb juice for every 1 cup (250 mL) of marinade, dressing or sauce and up to 1/4 cup (50 mL) in soups, stocks and stews — start with less and add to taste; the juice of herbs is more potent than the fresh leaf.

TINCTURES

It's not clear when tinctures came into popular use. Nicholas Culpeper, writing in the 17th century, makes no mention of them in his *Compleat Herbal*, although he does give directions for making fourteen different preparations, including pills. But, by the 19th century, there were hundreds of tinctures listed in the *United States Pharmacopoeia* (the official annual listing by the U.S. Government of pharmaceutical raw materials and recipes in regular use).

Tinctures are still useful for the herbalist because they offer potent, concentrated doses of the healing properties of the herbs from which they are made. They are used in small amounts, usually measured in drops, and added to water or clear herbal tea to be sipped slowly, or they can be applied externally as compresses.

To Make a Tincture

Herbs: Most medicinal herbs growing in the wild or in the garden work well in tinctures. Dandelion, burdock, valerian, ginseng and echinacea roots; alfalfa, hyssop and thyme leaves; and chamomile flowers work well in tinctures.

Alcohol: Use any fine grain spirits such as brandy, vodka or gin. Never use poisonous rubbing (isopropyl) alcohol or methyl (wood) alcohol.

4 oz	finely cut fresh herb	100 g
2 cups	alcohol	500 mL

1. In a large jar or jug with a tight-fitting lid, put herb leaves, petals or chopped root. Pour alcohol over herb to cover, seal jar. Shake well and leave in a warm, dark place for 14 days, shaking once or twice daily.
2. Strain into a dark glass bottle with tight-fitting lid, label and store in a cool, dark place for 2 to 5 years.

Makes: 2 cups (500 mL)

To take in a drink: count drops as they fall from a dropper or spoon into a cup of herbal tea or plain, filtered water. The usual dose is 5 to 10 drops, two to three times per day.

To use in cooking: Where fresh or dried ginseng, dandelion, burdock and echinacea root is called for in any of the recipes in this book, substitute 1 to 2 tsp (5 to 10 mL) of the tincture.

Add 1 tsp (5 mL) tincture to 2 cups (500 mL) vegetable stock.

As an immune-system booster, for short periods of time, tincture of echinacea may be taken in soups made with shiitake mushrooms and astragalus (follow the amounts given above). Take 3 to 4 cups (750 mL to 1 L) of the soup per day for 2 to 3 days.

SYRUPS

Mrs. Grieve, in *A Modern Herbal*, states that, "Almost from time immemorial, a Rob [a vegetable juice thickened by heat] has been made from the juice of Elderberries simmered and thickened with sugar, forming an invaluable cordial for colds and coughs...To make Elderberry Rob, 5 lb. of fresh, ripe, crushed berries are simmered with 1 lb. of loaf sugar and the juice evaporated to the thickness of honey. It is cordial, aperient and diuretic. One or two tablespoonsful mixed with a tumblerful of hot water, taken at night, promotes perspiration and is demulcent to the chest. The Rob when made can be bottled and stored for the winter. Herbalists sell it ready for use."

Fresh juice keeps only a couple of days and boiling the juice with sugar enabled herbalists to keep the resulting "rob" or syrup for long periods of time without refrigeration. It also had the added benefit of making the herbs easy to take.

Knowing what we now do about sugar, it is difficult to recommend that we take large quantities of syrup. However, if used with the intention of being a medicinal preparation and taken in small amounts, syrups do still have a place in herbal medicine and cooking.

To Make a Syrup

Herbs: Calendula, chamomile, and lavender flowers; and peppermint, thyme, sage, parsley and hyssop leaves are appropriate for making syrups. (To make a syrup from roots, follow directions on next page for making crystallized roots.)

1 cup	chopped fresh leaves or flowers	250 mL
1 quart	water	1 L
3 cups	sugar	750 mL
1/2 cup	honey	125 mL

1. In a stock pot, place herbs and add water; cover with a lid. Bring to a boil; reduce heat and simmer gently 20 minutes.

2. Strain off herb; return tea to pot. Add sugar and gently boil with lid on, about 1 hour, until mixture thickens and reaches about 200° F (95° C).

3. Remove from heat, stir in honey. Pour into sterilized jars.

Makes: 4 cups (1 L)
Substitute: corn syrup for honey

How to Use Syrups in Cooking

Use healing syrups in dishes where honey or maple syrup are called for. Add to custards, sauces and compotes in place of sugar. Use as a sweetener for herbal teas, cold drinks such as lemonade or iced mint tea, and hot drinks like mulled wine or apple cider.

COUGH SYRUP

This recipe may be cut in half.

1/2 cup	chopped fresh peppermint leaves	125 mL
1/4 cup	chopped fresh coltsfoot flowers or leaves	50 mL
1/4 cup	chopped fresh thyme leaves	50 mL
2 tbsp	chopped fresh hyssop leaves and flowers	25 mL
2 tbsp	chopped fresh horehound leaves and flowers	25 mL
1	2-inch (5 cm) piece each of ginger, licorice and ginseng root, crushed	1
4 cups	water	1 L
2 cups	sugar	500 mL
1/2 cup	honey	125 mL

1. In a stock pot, place herbs and add water; cover with a lid. Bring to a boil; reduce heat and simmer gently 20 minutes.

2. Strain off herbs; return tea to pot. Add sugar and gently boil about an hour, until mixture thickens and reaches about 200° F (95° C).

3. Remove from heat, stir in honey. Pour into sterilized jars, store in refrigerator.

Makes: 4 cups (1 L)
Substitute: sage for hyssop leaves and flowers
Omit: horehound if not available
Dose: 1 tbsp (5 mL) taken when needed to soothe coughs. Or mix 1 tbsp (15 mL) with 1/4 cup (50 mL) apple cider or medicinal vinegar and sip over a period of 2 to 4 hours.

CRYSTALLIZED ROOTS

Candied ginger has been a favorite of people around the world for years. Try this traditional method with other medicinal roots such as dandelion, burdock, licorice, ginseng (if you can get fresh roots) and echinacea.

2 cups	sliced (1/4-inch [5 mm] thick) root, skin on	500 mL
	filtered water	
1 1/2 cups	granulated sugar	375 mL
Half	lemon, sliced	Half
1 cup	light corn syrup	250 mL
1/2 cup	granulated sugar, if desired	125 mL

Day 1: In a large non-reactive saucepan, cover sliced or cubed root with water. Cover with lid and slowly bring to a boil over medium heat (this could take an hour). Reduce heat to medium-low and simmer gently for an hour. Add 1/2 cup (125 mL) of the sugar, stir well, and return to a boil. Remove the pan from the heat. Let the mixture stand, covered, at room temperature overnight.
Day 2: With lid on, bring the mixture to a boil, reduce the heat to medium-low, and simmer gently for 15 minutes. Stir in the lemon and corn syrup. Simmer, uncovered, 15 minutes longer, stirring occasionally. Remove the pan from the heat, cover, and let the mixture stand overnight.
Day 3: Bring the mixture to a boil again, stirring often. Stir in 1/2 cup (125 mL) of the sugar, bring to a boil, reduce the heat, and simmer gently, uncovered, for 30 minutes. Stir in the remaining 1/2 cup (125 mL) of sugar and bring to a boil. Remove the pan from the heat, cover, and let stand overnight.
Day 4: Remove lemon slices, bring the mixture to a boil. When the syrup drops heavily from the side of a spoon and the root is translucent (after about 20 minutes), remove the pan from the heat. At this point you can transfer root and syrup directly to a sterilized jar (I prefer this way of storing the roots — it keeps them moist and soft). Or pour off the syrup (save for other uses) and dry the root slices on a rack over waxed paper overnight and when well dried, roll in granulated sugar and store in tightly covered glass jars.
Makes: about 2 1/2 cups (625 mL) with syrup about 1 1/2 cups (375 mL) dried, without syrup
Store: in refrigerator

How to Use Candied Roots in Cooking

Use candied roots as you would fresh, pass as after-dinner delicacies, chop and drizzle with the syrup over desserts, hot cereal and fresh fruit.

VINEGARS

In 1665, the Great Plague ravaged London with as many deaths as 7,000 per week. Four thieves brewed up a potent vinegar that protected them while they plundered the dead bodies of plague victims. Ingredients of this magic brew included: rue, sage, mint, wormwood, rosemary, lavender flowers, camphor, cinnamon, nutmeg, cloves, garlic and Calamus aromaticus mixed into red wine vinegar. It is said that the "Four Thieves' Vinegar" saved them from the deadly disease.

Vinegar was in use long before the 17th century. Residue of vinegar in an Egyptian vessel dates its use as far back as 3000 BC. In 1394 winemakers in France established a guild of professional vinegar makers, the Corporatif des Maitres-Vinaigriers d'Orléans. Balsamic vinegar, from the province of Modena in Italy, has been made since the Middle Ages when it was named *balsamico* (a balsam) because of its esteemed medicinal properties. As a means of preserving the medicinally active components of herbs, vinegar was (and still is) an excellent tool. Alone or fortified with antiseptic herbs (such as thyme, garlic, lavender, sage, and hyssop), vinegar would have been an effective antiseptic.

Vinegar is produced in two stages. First, the sugars in fruit juice are converted into alcohol, then bacteria convert the alcohol to acetic acid. We make vinegars now almost entirely for their flavor for culinary purposes. But without knowing it, every time we make tarragon vinaigrette from homemade tarragon vinegar, we are enjoying not only the fragrance and taste of this fine culinary herb, but also the active medicinal properties it holds.

To Make a Healing Vinegar

A good-quality, natural white wine vinegar is the best one to use for culinary herbed vinegars. For medicinal purposes, herbalists recommend organic cider vinegar. Because this can overpower the herbs, it is better to use more herbs than less when making herbed medicinal vinegars. Taste vinegars as they are steeping and gauge the length of time by the flavor. If a vinegar is too strong, simply add more vinegar, but if it is too weak, it is not easy to add more herbs.

1	bunch herbs, slightly bruised	1
1 cup+	organic cider vinegar	250 mL+

1. In a clean glass bottle or ceramic crock, pack herbs.

2. Pour vinegar over the herbs and leave a 1-inch (2.5 cm) headspace. Close container with a cork (do not use metal lids, which may corrode and seep into the vinegar). Place in a sunny window for 2 weeks, turning frequently.

3. Strain into fresh clean jars, label and store in a dark, cool place.

HEALING VINEGAR COMBINATIONS

The flavor and medicinal effects of vinegar combinations are endless. Some suggestions for herbs to use in making healing vinegars are listed below. Amounts given are meant to be combined with one quart (1 L), more or less, of vinegar. Follow directions for making healing vinegar, above.

2 cups	rose petals,	500 mL
2 tbsp	cloves	25 mL
1 cup	chamomile flowers	250 mL
1 cup	elder flowers	250 mL
1 cup	lavender	250 mL
2 cups	calendula petals	500 mL
1	1-inch (2.5 cm) piece each ginseng and ginger, chopped	1
4 to 6	whole cayenne peppers	4 to 6
10 to 12	cloves whole garlic, peeled and crushed	10 to 12
2 cups	ginkgo leaves	500 mL
2 bunches	rosemary	2

ELDERBERRY VINEGAR

Add this healing vinegar to cough syrups; use in place of raspberry vinegar in vinaigrettes, sauces and dressings.

8 cups	elderberries, cleaned and picked over	2 L
1 quart	white wine vinegar	1 L
3 1/2 cups	sugar	875 mL

1. In a large bowl, mash the berries. Pour vinegar over and allow to stand for 24 to 36 hours, covered with a clean tea towel.

2. Strain through a jelly-bag, muslin or cheese-cloth. Allow to drain slowly for up to 24 hours (if you press on the fruit while it is draining, the vinegar will be cloudy).

3. Pour juice into a large non-reactive stock pot or preserving pan. Stir in the sugar, bring to a boil, adjust heat, allow to simmer for about 15 minutes. Pour into clean bottles with cork lids, label and store in a dark, cool place.

Makes: 6 cups (1.5 L)

How to Use Medicinal Vinegars in Cooking

Substitute medicinal vinegar in all recipes that call for regular vinegar. Add 2 to 4 tbsp (25 to 50 mL) to sauces, soups, stocks, stews.

OILS

Herbalists extract active plant ingredients in oil, for external use in massage oils, creams, salves, and ointments. For medicinal, external use only, any vegetable oil is suitable, with almond oil recommended for face and hand applications. Comfrey, St. John's wort, calendula, chamomile, rosemary and chickweed are all herbs that are well-used topical medicinal oils.

Cooks extract flavor from herbs in oil to enhance sauces and stir-fries. It seems natural that culinary oils should be made first with the healing properties of herbs in mind, then according to flavor. Healing herbs that impart superb flavor include rosemary, lavender, garlic, cayenne, thyme and sage.

Polyunsaturated fats, while they do reduce cholesterol, also reduce levels of "good" cholesterol — high density lipoprotein (HDL). HDL eliminates "bad" cholesterol (LDL, low density lipoprotein) from the cells and carries it towards elimination. Monounsaturated oils are now the most favored oils because they increase HDL while reducing artery-clogging LDL. For this reason, all recipes in this book call for a good quality olive oil.

Olive Oil Terms

Virgin Olive Oil: The term "virgin" is applied to an oil that has been obtained from olives without using heat during extraction: the olives are not subjected to any treatment other than washing, filtering, decanting or centrifuging.

Cold Pressed: Refers to the old method of collection, when the first olives through the press were pressed slowly, before the press heated up with its own friction. Now, new technology allows olives to be processed continuously without heat.

Extra Virgin: In olive oils labeled "extra virgin," only 1 percent acidity is allowed. Extra virgin olive oil has the highest quality taste and aroma; use it in vinaigrettes and sauces where the flavor will shine through.

Olive Oil: Oils labeled 100% olive oil are a blend of refined virgin olive oil and virgin or extra virgin; use them for sautés and stir-fries.

To Make a Healing Oil

All oils, including those labeled "light," deliver the

same amount of energy in our diet — 90 calories (370 kilojoules) per 2 tsp (10 mL). "Light" refers to the flavor, not the number of calories (kilojoules) in the oil.

| 1 bunch | herbs, slightly bruised | 1 |
| 1 cup+ | olive oil | 250 mL+ |

1. In a clean glass bottle or ceramic crock, pack herbs.
2. Pour oil over the herbs and leave a 1-inch (2.5 cm) headspace. Close container with a cork or lid. Place in a sunny window for 2 weeks, turning frequently.
3. Strain into fresh, clean jars; label and store in refrigerator.

HEALING OIL COMBINATIONS

Cooking with oils infused with medicinal herbs means that an extra hit of those healing qualities will be given to the food each time they are used. Make up your own combinations according to personal requirements. Follow directions for making healing oil, above. Suggested combinations:
• 4 sprigs peppermint; 3 cloves garlic, smashed; 2 tbsp (25 mL) cumin seeds; 2-inch (5 cm) piece each turmeric, chopped and cinnamon, crushed; 1 tbsp (15 ml) each whole cloves and allspice berries
• 10 sprigs thyme; 3 cloves garlic, smashed; 2-inch (5 cm) piece ginseng, chopped; 4 sticks astragalus
• 10 calendula flowers; 2-inch (5 cm) piece each ginger, chopped and licorice root, crushed

How to Use Medicinal Oils in Cooking

Substitute medicinal oils in all recipes where oil is required.

SOUPS

Eowtes of Flessh (Herb Soup)

Take borage, colewort (cabbage), lang-debuf (bugloss), persel (parsley), betes (beets), orach, violet, savory and fenkel (fennel), cut into small pieces and cast them in gode broth, seeth (boil) them and serve them forth.
From *The Forme of Cury*, 1390

All societies use the technique of simmering plants in water for nourishment.

Gentle, healing soups are a staple, next to rice, in Chinese kitchens. Made from nourishing vegetables and herbs such as astragalus and poria, they are taken morning, noon and night. In *The Food Book*, James Trager notes, "Mushroom and barley soup, made of imported dried mushrooms...is a Jewish favorite, as is potato soup. So are cold soups like borscht, a purée, hot or cold, of shredded (or finely sliced) beets with thick sour cream; *shav*, made from finely chopped sorrel (or sour grass) blended with sour cream; and fruit soup made of various fruits stewed in their own juices." The French have their soupe *bonne femme* and *pistou*, clear broth or vegetable soup topped with pesto. A French chef at the Ritz Carlton Hotel in New York invented vichyssoise, a cold potato and leek soup, in 1910 to celebrate the opening of the the roof garden. According to Trager, "Boston's... clam chowder got its name from *la chaudiere*, the enormous copper pot of early French coastal villages. Returning fishermen used to toss parts of their catch into *la chaudiere* and the community would make a soup to feast the safe return of the men from the sea." No matter the name or the country of origin, long-simmering soups made with fresh organic produce and whole grains deliver the goodness of plants and herbs, along with a warm sense of well-being.

Soup Stocks

The backbone of whole, fresh cooking is a good stock and many of the recipes in this book call for vegetable stock. In ideal kitchens, every few days, a new batch is made to be kept in the refrigerator up to 2 days or frozen for longer storage. However, very good canned organic, low sodium stocks are available at whole food and health/alternative stores.

HEALING VEGETABLE STOCK

Roasting the vegetables lends a rich taste and color to the stock. If time does not permit roasting, simply sauté onion, garlic and leek in the stockpot first, then add all other items. Or, for an extremely easy stock, omit the oil and toss all ingredients into the pot, simmer for 1 hour and strain.

1	large onion, quartered	1
4	cloves garlic, peeled	4
1	leek, trimmed, washed, cubed	1
2 tbsp	olive oil	25 mL
8 cups	water	2 L
Half	green cabbage, quartered	Half
1	stalk celery, coarsely chopped	1
1 each:	carrot, apple coarsely chopped	1
1	whole dried cayenne pepper	1
1 cup	coarsely chopped broccoli stems	250 mL
1	bay leaf	1
5	whole allspice berries	5

5	each: cloves, peppercorns	5
1	bunch fresh thyme, alfalfa	1
2 sprigs	fresh sage	2
3	pieces astragalus, if available	3
1- to 2-inch	pieces ginger, ginseng, burdock, dandelion root	2.5 to 5 cm

1. On a baking sheet, toss onion, garlic and leek with olive oil. Roast 30 to 40 minutes at 400° F (200° C), stirring once, until browned and crisp.
2. Meanwhile, in a large stockpot, bring water to a boil. Add all other ingredients; adjust heat to simmer and add roasted vegetables when browned.
3. Simmer 45 to 90 minutes; strain vegetables and discard. Refrigerate vegetable stock in jars with tight-fitting lids or freeze in 2-cup (500 mL) portions in freezer bags.

Makes: 8 cups (2 L)

Omit: any ingredient, if not available, except onion, garlic, cabbage

Add: To boost the potassium level of this stock, add sea herbs (such as dulse, kelp, *nori*), alfalfa, chamomile, burdock root, dandelion root, nettles, plantain leaves.

To boost the calcium level of this stock, add sea vegetables (such as *arame*, *hijiki*, kelp, *kombu*, *nori*, *wakame*), burdock root, dandelion greens, lambs-quarter, garlic, broccoli

Antioxidant herbs such as thyme or hyssop may also be added.

Note: While onion, garlic and cabbage remain central to this basic vegetable stock, all of the other ingredients are optional. Add parsnips, mushrooms, rutabaga or fennel if you have them or omit leek, the roots and astragalus if you don't have them. Potatoes and beets are not suitable for this stock, however beet tops and spinach are. The point is that cooking with this nutrient-rich broth boosts the nutrients in dishes where it is used. Use it in every recipe (even bread) that calls for water.

SEASONINGS

Seasonings are, by definition, "that which gives relish to food; anything that increases pleasure." Seasonings may be herbs or spices, or a blend of both, and are usually dried, powdered and added to food before, during and after cooking.

To Make Healing Seasonings

Dry herbs as instructed on page 36. Store in airtight tins or dark-colored jars. Blend small quantities of healing seasonings at a time. Mix equal amounts or in amounts as directed and grind to a powder using a mortar and pestle, food processor or blender. Divide in half and keep a small amount at the stove and at the table.

Antibiotic Seasonings

Natural antibiotics help the immune system work better, help to prevent infection without dangerous side effects and compensate for some of the side effects of prescription antibiotics.

SOME NATURAL ANTIBIOTICS FROM PLANT SOURCES

garlic	thyme
echinacea	hypericum (St. John's Wort)
goldenseal	*reishi*, *maitake* and shiitake mushrooms
calendula	capsicum (cayenne pepper)
licorice	Essiac® (includes sheep sorrel, burdock,
astragalus	slippery elm)
horseradish	juniper berries
nasturtium	red clover flowers

To make an antibiotic seasoning: start with dried flowerheads, roots, leaves or stems of the plant. Unless given specific amounts, mix equal amounts of two or three herbs listed above and pulverize in a mortar and pestle, blender or food processor. Store in a dark-colored jar in a cool, dry place.

SWEET ANTIBIOTIC SEASONING

1/4 cup	echinacea petals + leaves	50 mL
1/4 cup	calendula petals	50 mL
1	1-inch (2.5 cm) piece licorice root	1
1	whole clove	1

Makes: 3/4 cup (175 mL)

SAVORY ANTIBIOTIC SEASONING

1/4 cup	echinacea petals and leaves	50 mL
2	dried mushrooms	2
2	cayenne peppers	2
3 tbsp	thyme leaves	45 mL
3 tbsp	rosemary leaves	45 mL

Makes: 1/2 cup (125 mL)

To use as a salt substitute: blend either of the antibiotic seasonings above with 1 tbsp (15 mL) finely chopped dulse for every 1/4 cup (50 mL) seasoning.

To Use Antibiotic Seasonings in Cooking:

For best results as a preventative, use antibiotic seasonings at the table as an after cooking seasoning.

Sweet antibiotic seasoning: blend with stevia or sweet cicely and use as a natural sweetener for teas and other hot and cold beverages; blend 1 tbsp (15 mL) with curry spices and use in cooking — chicken, stir-fried vegetables, rice dishes and lentils.

Savory antibiotic seasoning: blend 1 tbsp (15 mL) with fresh garlic and use in cooking — soups, stews, stir-fries.

To use either of the above antibiotic seasonings as a rub for roasted or grilled vegetables, poultry or fish, blend 2 tbsp (25 mL) with 2 fresh cloves of garlic or 1/4 cup (50 mL) prepared mustard or healing syrup.

IMMUNE-BOOSTING SEASONING

Blend equal amounts of dried chopped echinacea root, dried chopped ginseng root and crushed astragalus sticks. Grind small amounts as needed, store in dark glass bottles at the table and at the stove.

MEMORY-BOOSTING SEASONING

Grind the herbs before measuring for this blend.

1 tbsp	scullcap (*scutellaria spp*)	15 mL
1 tbsp	ginger	15 mL
2 tbsp	rosemary	15 mL
3 tbsp	ginkgo (*ginkgo biloba*)	45 mL

1. Blend thoroughly; store in dark glass bottles at the table and at the stove.

Makes: about 1/2 cup (125 mL)

HEALING CURRY PASTE

1	2-inch (2.5 cm) piece cinnamon, crushed	1
1 tbsp	coriander seeds	15 mL
2 tsp	cumin seeds	10 mL
8	fresh green chilies, seeded, chopped	8
4	cloves garlic, chopped	4
2 tbsp	fresh chopped thyme	25 mL
1 tbsp	turmeric	15 mL
1 tbsp	green tea leaves	15 mL
2 tsp	anchovy paste	10 mL

1. In a small skillet or wok, heat cinnamon, coriander and cumin seeds for 1 to 2 minutes.

2. Using a pestle and mortar or food processor, crush toasted cinnamon and seeds.

3. Add remaining ingredients and pound or mix to a smooth paste. Store in an airtight jar in the refrigerator for up to 4 weeks. Use 1 tbsp (15 mL) in cooking as you would curry powder.

Makes: about 1/2 cup (125 mL)

Substitute: 8 dried chilies for fresh (yield will decrease); 2 whole anchovies for paste.

WINES

While the history and discovery of wine is not well-documented, we do know that the Egyptians made wine 5,000 years ago and that by 2,500 BC, Greeks and Romans spread its use to all parts of the Mediterranean and Europe. As a beverage, wine was safer than water. Louis Pasteur claimed, "Wine can be considered with good reason as the most healthful and the most hygienic of all beverages." Now, recent studies have explored the ways wine components may serve as antioxidants and have other potentially beneficial effects.

Those studies report that proanthocyanidins (OPCs), a group of compounds having antioxidant effects 20 to 50 times as powerful as vitamins C and E, are mostly concentrated in the seeds, skins and barks of plants. Because the skin is used in red wine, it is considered to have anti-aging effects and may lower LDL ("bad") cholesterol. Wine may be considered part of a healthy lifestyle when consumed moderately (i.e. one glass) with the main meal of the day. Wine is not recommended for people with a history of alcoholism, hypertension, liver disease, smoking, diabetes, obesity, or peptic ulcers.

There are two ways to enjoy the medicinal benefits of herbs through the use of wine. The first requires a basic knowledge of winemaking and the equipment that is essential to making wines at home. Any herb such as thyme, tarragon, rosemary, parsley, mint, calendula or dandelion can be used to make wine. Recipes using local fruits, flowers and herbs in what is commonly referred to as "country" wine are found in winemaking books. Experimentation with the different herbs is required after a basic skill level is achieved. I have made wine with lemon thyme and elderflower — both rendered an enjoyable product.

The other way to benefit from medicinal wine is easier, requires no special equipment and results are faster to achieve. Directions are simple: Place flowering herbs such as thyme, sage, rosemary, elder, mint, calendula (petals only), burdock root or dandelion flowers or root in a large, wide-mouthed glass jar that has an airtight lid. Pour organic red or white wine (organic hard or soft apple cider may also be used) over the herbs, cap and place the jar in a cool, dark place to allow the mixture to macerate for about 2 weeks. Strain off the herbs and discard. Bottle the liquid in green or brown bottles with corks or tight-fitting lids. Store between 40 and 50° F (5 and 10° C), out of light. Use any good organic red or white wine or apple cider. In both cases, the alcohol acts as a natural preservative for the medicinal properties of the herbs.

How to Use Healing Wines in Cooking

Substitute healing wine where vinegar is called for, especially in dressings and vinaigrettes. Use to add flavor to sauces, soups and stews and with fresh fruit. They can be used to tone down the bitter quality of tonics and other medicinal mixtures meant to be taken in small doses. The alcohol in wine will evaporate at 160° F (70° C), leaving only its flavor and medicinal qualities behind.

Healthy Cooking

More than anything else, our way of eating dictates our ability to resist disease. It is well known now that as stress increases in our lives, our immunity decreases. What is even more disturbing is that as our lives become more pressured, our ways of nourishing ourselves become more reliant upon fast, unnatural foods, foods that offer no help in building up our immune responses, so that we end up with a double whammy — high stress and poor nutrition.

You may find that when you begin to eat a whole-food diet, your body has difficulty in digesting and responds with slight cramping, gas and increased elimination. All these body functions will level out if you persist. In part, the reason for giving you the detailed information about the healing properties of both the foods and herbs is to motivate you to change your diet and give you reasons to stick to it. It's wonderful to be thinking about the anti-cancer benefits of mushrooms as you chop and prepare them for a rich brothy soup or risotto.

Phytochemistry — the identification, biosynthesis and metabolism of chemical constituents of plants and their effect on the body — is a dynamically growing field and there are already good books which outline the nature and function of each nutrient. Some of those books are listed in the bibliography of this book (page 180).

Healthy cooking, as already stated, means increasing our intake of foods with which we may need to introduce or re-acquaint ourselves. The richly complex multitude of substances in food and herbs working in concert with each other can be combined and eaten to keep us healthy.

Legumes

Dried peas, beans and lentils are called legumes because they are the seeds of plants that produce their seeds in pods. The term "legume" can mean the plant, the pods or the seeds. In Europe and Asia, the term "pulse" means fresh or dry edible leguminous seeds and is interchanged with the word legume. *Dal* is a Middle-East and Eastern term for a specific group of legumes which includes split peas, blackeyed peas, small black beans, mung beans and all types of lentils. The word *dal* also refers to a purée-style dish made from any of those legumes.

Many cultures cook with legumes and, from time to time, they have been thought of as "poor man's food." But their unrefined, high-protein, low-fat qualities have earned them respect as "fit food" as we enter the 21st century. Legumes offer an excellent source of soluble and insoluble dietary fiber in the form of gums, mucilages, and pectin. That, along with isoflavonoids, lignins, phytate and folic acid help to lower cholesterol, protect against colon and breast cancer, guard against heart disease and diverticulosis, and modulate blood-sugar levels. In addition, they offer a satisfying, low-fat source of complex carbohydrates.

High in B vitamins (except B12), 1 cup (250 mL) cooked beans equals 40 percent of the daily requirement of thiamine and B6 and one-quarter of the daily requirement of iron. Legumes are also an excellent source of calcium, phosphorus and potassium.

Legumes (except soybeans, which contain complete protein) are an excellent source of incomplete protein — meaning that they don't supply the body with all 8 essential amino acids, being low in methionine and high in lysine. They are often combined with whole grains and this combination is an excellent amino acid (complete protein) balance because whole grains are high in methionine and low in lysine. The legume/whole-grain combination is complementary, offering the body an excellent protein balance that can easily substitute for meat.

WHOLE AND ANCIENT GRAINS

The term "whole grains" means simply that — the three important parts of the grain are left intact, or whole. Whole grains are an extremely useful food as, being unrefined, they retain all the nutritional value of the bran and germ and add fiber to the diet. Refined grains, on the other hand, have been processed to remove the bran and germ, leaving only the starchy, least nutritious, fiber-stripped, bleached endosperm. Studies have proved that the processing and refinement of foods, especially grains, has led to modern degenerative diseases (colon cancer, diabetes, heart problems).

Whole grains supply complex carbohydrates to the body. They are complex because the whole seed package with its three major departments is intact. The outer layer, called bran, protects the grain's life force and nourishment. It contains fiber, minerals and protein. It is always removed in the refinement process. The largest part of the grain is the endosperm, which provides a storehouse of food in the form of carbohydrate for the seed when it starts to grow. The germ is the life-spark of the grain and is a rich source of protein, minerals and vitamins. Government nutritional guides recommend that we eat 5 to 12 servings of grain products each day and encourage us to choose whole grain products more often.

Actions: The nutrients and phytochemicals in whole grains combine to help prevent against colon cancer; halt the early stages of breast cancer; protect against cancer of the large intestine; have an antioxidant effect; ward off heart disease; fight obesity; and lower blood sugar levels.

Phytochemicals: In all, whole grains offer protein, carbohydrate, phytate, vitamin E, fiber (including lignins), and some B vitamins (thiamin, riboflavin, niacin, folacin), iron, zinc and magnesium.

SOY FOODS

Soybeans are the only known vegetable source of "complete protein," meaning that they contain all of the essential amino acids in the appropriate proportions essential for the growth and maintenance of body cells. In addition to being an excellent source of fiber, the fat in soybeans — 34% — is polyunsaturated, lower than animal fat in calories and rich in lenolenic and lenoleic fatty acids.

A group of flavonoids called isoflavones — including genistein, daidzein and glycitein — are abundant in soybeans and soy foods (a serving of tofu or a glass of soy milk contains therapeutic levels of these substances). Research has shown that isoflavones are powerful antioxidants that minimize cell damage from free radicals, block the damaging effects of hormonal or synthetic estrogens, and inhibit tumor cell growth. All of the effects of isoflavones combine to lower the risk of cancer and lower cholesterol by preventing its absorption from the gastrointestinal tract. Diets high in soy are documented as preventing cancers of the prostate, breast, uterus, lungs, colon, stomach, liver, pancreas, bladder and skin.

Other components found in soybeans are: saponins, which boost immunity, prevent infections and cancer, and lower cholesterol; phytic acid, an antioxidant also linked to cancer prevention; phytosterols which aid in the prevention of colon cancer; and omega-3 essential fatty acids, important to the immune system and for reducing the risk of heart disease, arthritis, and high blood pressure.

With all of the incredible, clinical and epidemiological studies — over 1,000 published studies since 1993 — it makes a lot of sense to include soybeans and soy foods in our diet, at the very least 3 times per week for prevention, once a day for more aggressive treatment.

Soybeans: Available in the whole, raw, dried state. Must be rehydrated in the same way that other legumes are soaked, then cooked. *To soak:* In a large saucepan, place washed beans covered with 2 inches (5 cm) water. Bring to the boil, reduce heat and boil 2 minutes. Leave the pan on the element and turn off the heat. Allow to stand 1 hour (or overnight). Discard soaking water and rinse beans. Soybeans have now been rehydrated and are ready to cook. Never use salt or other seasonings at the soaking stage.
To cook: In a large saucepan, place soaked, drained, rinsed beans. Cover with 2 inches (5 cm) fresh water. Cover pan, bring to boil, reduce heat and simmer for about 3 hours, until tender. Pressure cooking reduces the soaking and cooking time significantly (check manufacturer's instructions). Add salt or other seasonings only after soybeans are cooked (adding earlier causes beans to be tough).
Tofu: Also called "bean curd" or "soy cheese," tofu is one of the most versatile soy foods. It is a custard-like product made from heating soy milk. Tofu can be purchased as either "soft" or "firm," which has more water pressed from it. Tofu can be frozen (the color turns yellow and the texture is more chewy), marinated, stir-fried, used as cottage cheese, as sandwich spreads, or mixed with salads, soups and pastas.

Tempeh: Pronounced "tem-PAY," it is a mild, meaty-tasting, firm white cake made from fermenting cooked soybeans. Usually frozen, tempeh gives a chewy texture to vegetarian dishes and is a good substitute for ground beef in pasta sauce or chili. It can be fried, baked, broiled, grilled or simmered with vegetables in other dishes.

SPROUTS

For over 2,000 years, the Chinese have used sprouted seeds, grains and beans as a staple food. Sprouts are the first germinated form of seeds — baby plants — used as green vegetables within the first couple of weeks of life. Vitamins and minerals are concentrated, and more abundant in sprouts than in other greens. High in vitamins B and C, iron, bioflavonoids, and enzymes, they add flavor and nutrients to meals. For example, alfalfa sprouts have 210 mg of calcium compared with 122 mg in spinach. Enzymes, which facilitate growth and repair of tissue are more abundant in sprouts because they are extremely perishable and only found in living foods. Recent research from Johns Hopkins University School of Medicine in Baltimore has shown that broccoli sprouts contain from 20 to 50 times the concentration of sulforaphane, an anti-cancer compound, as found in the mature plants.

As a source of green, living nutrition, sprouts are an easy crop for all locations and all seasons, especially important in winter. While legumes (like alfalfa, adzuki beans and lentils) and grains (such as wheat, rye or barley) are the most commonly sprouted seeds, you can also try sprouting the seeds of chives, onions, sunflowers, flax, peas, mustard, radishes, lettuce, cabbage, ancient grains (like kamut, spelt, quinoa) and any of the culinary and medicinal herbs (such as basil, garlic, cress, dill, hyssop, sage, thyme). Seeds of plants with poisonous foliage (like tomatoes, rhubarb and peppers), as well as those that are toxic when eaten raw (such as lima and fava beans) should not be sprouted.

To Sprout Seeds

If not using one of several sprouting kits available, you will need a clean wide-mouthed quart glass jar and a piece of cheesecloth or clean linen tea towel. Rinse 2 to 4 tbsp (25 to 50 mL) organic seeds in a fine metal sieve or right in the jar. Cover the jar with a layer of cheesecloth, secured with a rubber band, and pour off the rinse water. Add 1 cup (250 mL) warm water and set the jar in a warm place, out of direct sunlight (on the counter or in a cupboard), for 8 to 12 hours. Next day, drain off the water (use in cooking if

desired) and rinse the seeds in the jar. Drain off the rinse water (from now on, the only water that will be added will be the rinse water). As the jar fills with sprouts, rinse them 2 to 3 times a day. Rinsing provides enough moisture to keep the seeds growing, adds oxygen and removes waste components. Tilt the jar upside down or at least on its side so that extra water from each rinse can drain off. When the sprouts have reached the desired length, remove from the jar and use immediately or store in the refrigerator in a covered container, no longer than 2 to 3 days.

To Use Sprouts

Use sprouts as you would lettuce in salads and sandwiches; add at the last minute to soups, stir-fried vegetables; in dips, sauces, dressings; add 1 cup (250 mL) per loaf of bread when adding the liquid ingredients.

NUTS AND SEEDS

To our hunter-gatherer forebears, nuts and seeds were an important part of their healthy, natural diet. Packed with a natural energy reserve for plants, nuts and seeds contain protein, vitamin E and fiber with about 80 percent of their calories from fat. Although the fat is polyunsaturated or monounsaturated which may actually help decrease blood-cholesterol levels, nuts and seeds should be used regularly, but in moderation.

In their natural state (unpeeled, unsalted, raw), they add nutrients to diets high in complex carbohydrates and low in other fats. Nuts contain linoleic acid and alpha-linolenic acid, two essential fatty acids that are associated with decreased risk of tumor formation and heart disease and are also essential for healthy skin, hair, glands, mucus membranes, nerves, and arteries. Essential fatty acids regulate cholesterol production, menstruation, and blood pressure, absorption of calcium and the body's lubricants.

Isoflavones and ellagic acid, which both help to protect against cancer, are abundant in nuts. Flax seeds are high in lignins, thought to block or suppress the growth of cancer cells.
Nuts: almonds, brazil nuts, cashews, chestnuts, ginkgo, hazelnuts, macadamia nuts, pecans, pine nuts, pistachio nuts, walnuts (not peanuts, which are actually legumes).
Seeds: flax, poppy, sesame, sunflower
To store: Harvested in the fall, the freshest selection is available from late fall through winter. Buy and store nuts in the shell and open just before using. Exposure to air, light or heat oxidizes some nutrients and makes the fat rancid.

For those of you who have my first cookbook, *Recipes from Riversong: Using Herbs in Lean Green Cooking*, you will notice some changes in the nature of the recipes in this book. For one thing, I've matured, taken a well-seasoned (excuse the pun), more confident approach to cooking with herbs. Where teaspoons were timidly used before, I'm adding handfuls of fresh and tablespoons of dried herbs in dishes that are rich in whole grains, legumes and fresh vegetables. Take my word for it, they can take the extra zip but, if you are just starting to explore the use of herbs in cooking, try half the amounts called for, then increase as your taste buds direct.

Another noticeable departure is the absence of sugar (except syrups and candied roots) and refined flour in all recipes. And while fresh fruit is part of a healthy diet, it is recommended that fruit be taken an hour to 30 minutes before meals, one to two hours after meals, or between meals to eliminate gas.

The recipes in this book are organized by season within each section because herbs, vegetables and fruits grow according to their own natural rhythm. There is a response within us to the ebb and flow of the seasons and if we listen to it, our diet will reflect our changing needs in symmetry with our environment. Eating seasonally means choosing fruits, vegetables and herbs when they are at their peak in our own gardens or at local farms. It means waiting for local strawberries and asparagus in the spring, planning meals around tomatoes and peppers in the fall and foregoing them in winter. And it means thinking about the effects of mass-produced foods grown with extremely toxic chemicals and harmful methods, with every trip to the supermarket.

In keeping with the seasons, spring, summer and fall recipes call for fresh herbs, readily available in our gardens and at market while winter recipes use dried herbs. If you are substituting dried herbs for fresh, use the following equation: 1 tbsp (15 mL) fresh herbs = 1 tsp (5 mL) dried herbs.

Healthy food begins with healthy ingredients. Poisons and synthetic chemicals in the form of pesticides, herbicides and fertilizers cause cancer. Organic food is grown without chemicals and provides human nourishment at the same time as it protects the soil for future generations. The recipes in this book are designed to be made with organic ingredients. Thus, the peel is left on most fruit (such as pears, apples) and all vegetables (except eggplant and other thick-skinned varieties). If you find you must use non-organic ingredients, peel all fruit and vegetables and wash greens in water with a few drops of a non-toxic soap.

Fatty acids obtained from natural whole foods such as nuts, seeds, olives, avocados, fish and poultry are good sources of dietary fats. The three fatty acids considered to be essential to our health are omega-6 linoleic, omega-3 linolenic and gamma linolenic acids. Cooking with fats is still desirable in some recipes and while the *amount* of fat may be reduced, the *kind* of fat is even more important to our health. The most stable cooking oil is olive oil and for this reason, it is used in all recipes where heating is required. Cold filtered, virgin olive oil is the best oil to use in health smart recipes. Butter is the only other heat stable fat and is used in those recipes where its unique flavor is important to the dish. Never use margarine. Use polyunsaturated fats such as soybean, corn, safflower, flax and sunflower only when the recipe does not call for it to be heated.

Salt is not called for in the list of ingredients as it is recommended that foods be cooked without it. Directions to "season to taste" are given in the recipe instructions and that is your clue to add a salt substitute or a small amount of salt and pepper if you must. See "Healing Seasonings," pages 43-44, for salt substitutes to use in cooking and at the table.

While a small amount of animal protein, once or twice per week is acceptable, our North American diet is still very reliant on red meat. As our collective consciousness is raised about healthy eating and healthy food, we begin to question how animals are raised and the implications for land use. For these reasons and to suit the growing number of people who have made the decision to exclude meat from their diet, the recipes in this book are meat-free. However, you will find instructions on how to add meat to those dishes where it would be appropriate.

Substitutions are included with each recipe due to the fact that some ingredients may not be available to all people, and because, in the end, cooking is a personal endeavor. To put your own stamp on these recipes would be the greatest compliment you could give to me.

Eating live, whole foods is important to health and for this reason, canned foods are not called for in these recipes except in the following cases: tomatoes (for winter use), cooked legumes (beans, peas, lentils), and vegetable stock. Find a good health/alternative store near you and use it often. Along with many whole, live foods, it will carry organic canned products that are salt- and sugar-free.

Most importantly, the recipes are intended for you to enjoy!

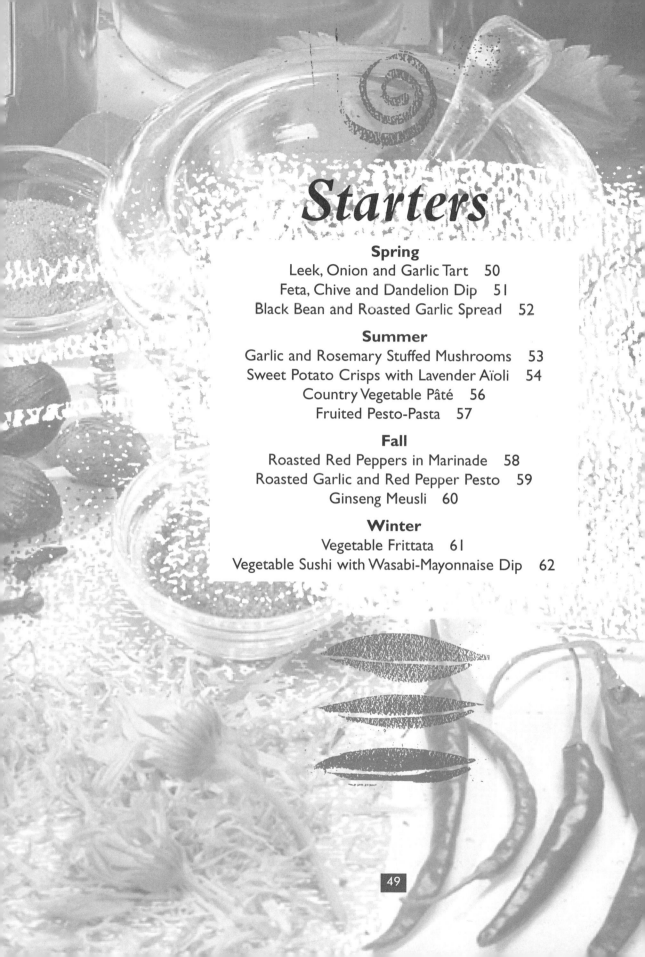

Starters

Leek, Onion and Garlic Tart

Serves 6

TIP

Using a springform pan makes serving easier because the sides can be removed. Serve hot or at room temperature. Slice in thin wedges for first course or use larger servings for a vegetable side dish.

VARIATIONS

Substitute: Regular potatoes or 1/2 acorn or butternut squash for sweet potatoes.

Rites of Spring (1)
The Druid Spring Equinox, meán Earraigh, was celebrated around March 21st, when night is equal to day in length. Rituals originating from the ancient Druids would have included eggs — symbols of rebirth, fertility and immortality — which were painted with symbols and pictures of what one wished to manifest in the coming year, then buried in the earth. Sacred hilltops were visited and picnics of figs, figcakes, cider and ale were part of the pleasures of spring. Figs are a symbol of fertility, with the leaf symbolizing the male, and the fruit representing the female element.

Preheat oven to 375° F (190° C)
10-inch (3 L) springform pan *or* round tart pan
or shallow baking dish, buttered

Base

3 cups	thinly sliced unpeeled potatoes	750 mL
1 cup	thinly sliced peeled sweet potatoes	250 mL
3 tbsp	honey mustard	45 mL
2 tbsp	olive oil	25 mL

Topping

1/4 cup	sliced leek, white part only	50 mL
4	cloves garlic, slivered	4
3 cups	sliced onions	750 mL
2 tbsp	olive oil	25 mL
3 tbsp	chopped fresh basil	45 mL
1/4 cup	freshly grated Parmesan cheese	50 mL

1. In a large bowl, toss potatoes with mustard and 2 tbsp (25 mL) oil. Spread in bottom of prepared pan. Press potatoes with the back of a spoon to compress. Season to taste with salt and pepper.

2. Spread leek and garlic evenly over potato base, then onions over top. If desired, season to taste with salt. Drizzle with oil. Bake in preheated oven for 40 minutes or until potatoes are tender and onions are golden. Sprinkle with basil and cheese; bake for another 5 minutes or until cheese has melted. Allow to stand for at least 10 minutes before serving.

Feta, Chive and Dandelion Dip

**Makes 2 1/3 cups
(575 mL)**

TIP

Use this creamy, low-fat spread/dip as a tasty substitute for sour cream on toasted bagels or baked potatoes.

If the yogurt is reduced to less than 1 1/3 cups (325 mL), add whey to reach the required volume.

VARIATIONS

Substitute: Fresh chopped green onions for chives; Spinach or lettuce for dandelion leaves; Calendula petals for dandelion petals.

Omit: Dandelion petals if not available; Cucumber if desired.

Rites of Spring (2)

Easter Day falls between March 21st and April 21st, the date still being calculated according to the first full moon of spring. Our rather tame Easter is linked with pagan cults of the Saxon spring goddess, Eostre, when single human sacrifices (usually young maidens) were made to ensure the lives of the whole community. Chrisitanity depicts Christ as a sacrificial lamb and modern Easter dinners often include lamb as a symbol of that sacrifice. Rosemary is used for remembrance, as it is the herb that represents the blue robes of the Virgin Mary.

2 cups	plain yogurt	500 mL
Half	English cucumber	Half
1 cup	crumbled feta cheese	250 mL
1/4 cup	chopped fresh chives	50 mL
1/4 cup	chopped fresh dandelion leaves	50 mL
1/4 cup	dandelion petals	50 mL
2	cloves garlic, minced	2

1. Measure yogurt into a sieve lined with cheesecloth set over a bowl. Allow to drain for 3 hours or until yogurt is reduced to 1 1/3 cups (325 mL).

2. Scrub cucumber (leave the peel on if organic) and shred into a sieve. Let stand for 30 minutes. Rinse, then squeeze lightly, discarding liquid.

3. Combine reduced yogurt, cucumber, feta cheese, chives, dandelion leaves, dandelion petals and garlic. Stir to mix well. If desired, season to taste with salt and pepper. Store in the refrigerator for up to 2 days.

Black Bean and Roasted Garlic Spread

Makes 2 cups (500 mL)

TIP

Black turtle beans give a smooth texture to this healing spread.

VARIATIONS

Substitute: Red wine or healing vinegar for balsamic vinegar.

	Preheat oven to 375° F (190° C) Small casserole dish with lid	
4	whole garlic heads	4
1/2 tbsp	olive oil	7 mL
1	can (19 oz [540 mL]) black beans	1
1 tbsp	olive oil	15 mL
2 tsp	balsamic vinegar	10 mL

1. Slice 1/4 inch (5 mm) off the top of each garlic head. Remove outer loose skin. Place each head cut-side up in casserole dish. Drizzle with 1/2 tbsp (7 mL) oil. Cover and bake in preheated oven for 40 to 45 minutes or until cloves are very soft. Remove from oven and allow to cool.

2. Meanwhile, place black beans in a food processor or blender. When garlic is cool enough to handle, squeeze cloves from heads into the food processor. Process until smooth. With the motor running, add 1 tbsp (15 mL) olive oil and vinegar; process until combined. If desired, season to taste with salt and pepper. Store in the refrigerator for up to 3 days.

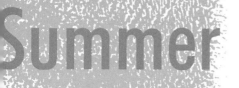
Summer

Garlic and Rosemary Stuffed Mushrooms

Serves 4

TIP

Use four portobello mushrooms in this recipe as a dramatic first course appetizer or, if served with a salad, as a light lunch.

The stuffing can be prepared up to 6 hours ahead and refrigerated.

VARIATIONS

Substitute: 1 tbsp (15 mL) dried rosemary leaves for fresh rosemary; 1 tbsp (15 mL) pesto for the combination of rosemary, butter and Parmesan cheese.

	Preheat oven to 375° F (190° C) Baking pan, lightly greased	
16	large mushrooms, cleaned and patted dry, stems removed and set aside	16
2	cloves garlic	2
1	slice 2-day-old whole grain bread, torn into pieces	1
6	whole almonds	6
1/4 cup	fresh parsley leaves	50 mL
2 tbsp	fresh rosemary leaves	25 mL
1 tbsp	butter	15 mL
3 tbsp	freshly grated Parmesan cheese	45 mL

1. Place mushroom caps, stem-side up, on prepared baking sheet.

2. In a food processor or blender, process reserved mushroom stems, garlic, bread and almonds until finely ground. Add remaining ingredients and process until well combined. If desired, season to taste with salt and pepper. Divide evenly into mushroom caps; bake in preheated oven for 15 to 20 minutes or until golden.

Sweet Potato Crisps with Lavender Aïoli

TIP

The flavor of the lavender aïoli is set off by the sweet potatoes. If serving with a regular mayonnaise or dip, toss the herbs listed below with the potatoes in step 2 to give the crisps a richer flavor.

VARIATIONS

Add any one of: 1 clove garlic, minced; 2 tbsp (15 mL) fresh chopped rosemary or basil pesto; 1 tsp (5 mL) fresh chopped sage; 1 tsp (5 mL) cayenne pepper.

Makes about 1 1/4 cups (300 mL)

TIP

This gives just a hint of garlic. Add another egg to use as a very delicate sauce for summer vegetables. Serve over lightly steamed asparagus, green beans or beets, or use as a dip.

Aïoli thickens upon chilling. Keep only 1 or 2 days in the refrigerator.

Preheat oven to 375° F (190° C)
2 large baking sheets, greased

Sweet Potato Crisps

2	large sweet potatoes	2
3 tbsp	olive oil	45 mL

1. Peel potatoes and slice diagonally, to get elongated rounds. Keep the slices as thin as possible, about 1/8 inch (2 mm).

2. In a large bowl, toss potatoes with oil. Spread potato slices in a single layer on prepared baking sheets.

3. Place in preheated oven for 12 minutes or until light brown on bottom. Remove sheets, flip slices, return to oven and cook for another 7 to 15 minutes or until lightly brown and crisp. (Some crisps may cook faster than others; remove from oven as soon as they are done.) Season to taste with salt and pepper.

4. Allow crisps to cool on wire racks. Serve slightly warm or at room temperature with a dollop of aïoli (recipe follows).

Lavender Aioli

1 cup	olive oil	250 mL
6	cloves garlic, unpeeled and crushed	6
2	fresh lavender sprigs, leaves and flower, bruised	2
3	eggs, room temperature	3
1 tbsp	lemon juice	15 mL

1. In a small saucepan, gently heat oil with garlic and lavender over low heat for about 15 minutes. Remove from heat just before oil starts to bubble. Allow to cool to room temperature.

Substitute: Rosemary,
sage, thyme, tarragon or
savory for lavender.

2. With a sieve over a small bowl, strain lavender oil, pressing with a spoon to extract soft solids from the garlic and lavender. Discard herbs.

3. In a food processor or blender, process egg and lemon juice until well blended. With the motor running, add oil a few drops at a time, then in a thin, steady stream until all oil is absorbed and mixture has thickened. Season to taste with salt.

AÏOLI AND MAYONNAISE

Ail is the French word for garlic. Aïoli is a simple garlic and olive oil sauce that is very popluar in Provence. It is a thick, golden mayonnaise that uses a minimum of 2 garlic heads for every 2 cups (500 mL) of oil and no other flavoring except salt. Tradition dictated that Aïoli be made every Friday, a day of fasting when only this sauce — and, perhaps, anchovies, boiled potatoes, artichokes, tomatoes, green beans, carrots, black olives or hard cooked eggs (what we call Niçoise Salad) — were eaten. People in the Mediterranean area were enjoying aïoli or the Spanish ali-oli long before the eighteenth century when a more sophisticated form — mayonnaise — was invented in France.

Some historical reference to mayonnaise appears in stories about the Duc de Richelieu who captured the British-held Port Mahon, on the Mediterranean island of Minorca in 1756. Theories on the origins of the word mayonnaise are conflicting. Some believe it comes from the old French term for egg yolk, moyeu. Others suspect it is taken from bay-onnaise, after the southern French town of Bayonne, near the Spainish

border. Having first appeared in print in English in 1841, it would be another 100 years before Richard Hellmann, a New York delicatessen owner, made mayonnaise popular in the United States. In 1932, California-based Best Foods merged with Hellmans to form one nationwide mayonnaise company. Today, mayonnaise is the largest-selling sauce in the United States (2.9 pounds of commercial mayonnaise are consumed by each American every year).

Aïoli was made by hand using a mortar. The garlic was crushed with a pestle, the egg yolks and salt were pounded into the garlic and then the oil was added drop by drop and whisked or beaten with a wooden spoon until the aïoli thickened.

This proceedure was tedious, time-consuming and required a strong arm. Now, with the help of modern machines such as the blender and the food processor, aïoli and its relative, mayonnaise, are easy to make. When using a machine, use the whole egg instead of just the yolk because the protein in the white acts as a stabilizer, preventing the high speed of the machine's blades from breaking up the emulsion.

As a condiment, homemade mayonnaise is preferable to the commercial product which is made, by law, with at least 65% vegetable oil by weight, — as well as vinegar and/or lemon juice, egg yolk, salt, sweeteners, monosodium glutamate and preservatives. However, one tablespoon (15 mL) olive oil (or homemade aïoli or mayonnaise) delivers about 120 calories compared to 100 calories for commercial mayonnaise. But a tablespoon of aïoli gives you the concentrated punch of raw, fresh garlic and the goodness of the fresh egg. Use aïoli (and homemade mayonnaise) sparingly in place of commercial mayonnaise in all salads, sandwich mixes and spreads.

Caution: Raw eggs may contain salmonella and for this reason, homemade aioli and mayonnaise should always be refrigerated and stored for a maximum of 2 days. Never make salads or sandwiches with homemade aïoli or mayonnaise for picnics or outdoor meals as the heat encourages the growth of the dangerous bacteria.

Country Vegetable Pâté

Makes about 3 cups (750 mL)

Preheat oven to 400° F (200° C)
Large baking pan, greased

2	heads garlic, cloves peeled and left whole	2
1	onion, peeled and quartered	1
1	leek, white and tender green parts, cut into large chunks	1
15	small shiitake mushrooms *or* maitake mushrooms	15
1	zucchini, cut into large chunks	1
1	eggplant, cut into large chunks	1
2 tbsp	olive oil	25 mL
1/2 cup	packed dulse	125 mL
1/2 cup	hot water	125 mL
1/2 cup	chopped toasted pecans	125 mL
1/2 cup	cooked rice	125 mL
1/2 cup	whole wheat breadcrumbs	125 mL
2 tbsp	fresh chopped thyme	25 mL

1. In a large bowl, toss garlic, onion, leek, mushrooms, zucchini and eggplant with oil. If desired, season to taste with salt. Spread onto prepared baking pan. Bake in preheated oven for 20 to 30 minutes or until brown. Stir once or twice, removing vegetables as they are done. (The smaller vegetables will cook faster than the large ones.)

2. In a small bowl, cover dulse with water; allow to sit for 5 minutes. Drain, pressing lightly, reserving soaking liquid.

3. In a food processor or blender, combine roasted vegetables, drained dulse, pecans, rice, breadcrumbs and thyme. Pulse on and off until well mixed and chunky. If too dry to hold together, add a little reserved dulse soaking liquid until the consistency is right for spreading.

Summer

Fruited Pesto-Pasta

Serves 6

TIP

Any summer fruit works well in this refreshing appetizer. Use as a starting course or as a different main luncheon dish.

VARIATIONS

Substitute: Any summer fruit for the fruit called for in recipe; Any fresh pesto for calendula pesto.

8 oz	whole wheat pasta bows or shells	250 g
2 tbsp	olive oil	25 mL
2 tbsp	raspberry vinegar	25 mL
1/4 cup	CALENDULA PESTO (see recipe, page 172)	50 mL
1/2 cup	sliced strawberries	125 mL
1/2 cup	sliced peaches	125 mL
1/2 cup	sliced cherries	125 mL
1/2 cup	diced pears	125 mL

1. In a large pot of salted water, boil pasta for about 10 minutes or until tender but firm. Drain; transfer to a large bowl.

2. Meanwhile, in a jar with a tight-fitting lid, combine olive oil, vinegar and pesto. Shake well. Pour over pasta and toss; let cool.

3. Toss strawberries, peaches, cherries and pears with pasta. Serve within 2 hours at room temperature.

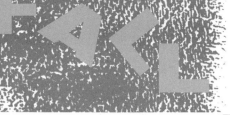

Roasted Red Peppers in Marinade

Makes 3 cups (750 mL)

TIP

Make this dish at the peak of pepper season when bushels are to be had at farmers' markets for the best price of the year. To make in quantity, they take time; but with many hands, it becomes a social event — an autumn tradition.

Peppers and marinade can be preserved in canning jars. Pack and seal according to the manufacturer's directions.

| | Preheat broiler
Baking pan | |
| --- | --- | --- |
| 4 | red bell peppers, halved and seeded | 4 |
| 1/3 cup | olive oil | 75 mL |
| 3 tbsp | balsamic vinegar | 45 mL |
| 4 | cloves garlic, thinly sliced lengthwise | 4 |

1. Place pepper halves cut-side down in baking pan. Place in preheated oven on top rack directly under heat for 5 to 8 minutes. Allow skin to char, turning pan often to ensure peppers are blackened evenly.

2. Meanwhile, whisk oil, vinegar and garlic together in a medium-sized bowl. Set aside.

3. Remove blackened peppers from oven. Cover with a clean towel and allow to cool. Remove the charred skin, which should slip off easily. Cut into 1-inch (2.5 cm) wide strips and place in bowl with oil mixture. Toss peppers well to coat evenly. Cover dish tightly with plastic wrap. Peppers should be allowed to marinate for at least 2 hours at room temperature and up to 3 days refrigerated.

Serving Suggestions

Spoon roasted peppers into four individual oven-proof dishes. Place one slice of creamy goat's cheese on top, bake at 350° F (180° C) for 5 to 10 minutes or until cheese is melted and peppers are bubbling. Serve warm as an appetizer.

Toss 2 cups (500 mL) roasted peppers with 1/2 cup (125 mL) chopped fresh basil and 4 servings cooked spaghetti.

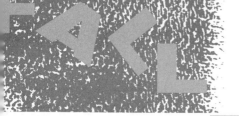

Roasted Garlic and Red Pepper Pesto

Makes 2 cups (500 mL)

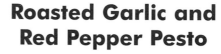

	Preheat oven to 375° F (190° C) Small casserole dish with lid	
2	heads garlic	2
1 tsp	olive oil	5 mL
2 cups	roasted red peppers, strained (see recipe, facing page, for technique)	500 mL
1 cup	fresh basil leaves	250 mL
1/4 cup	pine nuts	50 mL
1/4 cup	red pepper marinade (from recipe on facing page)	50 mL

1. Cut 1/4 inch (1 cm) off top of each garlic head. Remove outer loose skin and place each head in casserole dish, cut tops up. Drizzle with olive oil (1/2 tsp [2 mL] per head). Cover and bake in preheated oven for 40 to 45 minutes or until garlic is very soft. Remove from oven and allow to cool.

2. In a food processor or blender, squeeze garlic cloves from heads. Add red peppers, basil and pine nuts. Process until finely chopped. With motor running, add marinade. Process until smooth. Pack into clean jars and store in refrigerator. The pesto will keep one week in refrigerator and several months if frozen.

PRESERVING GARLIC

The traditional way to keep garlic for winter use has been to allow the buds to cure out of the ground, away from direct sunlight for 2 to 4 weeks. This allows the outer green leaf wrappers to dry, preventing mildew and fermentation. The bulbs are then stored in a cool, dark place. Many ways of braiding dried garlic have been developed and are still in use today; this being the best way to keep garlic.

Some old traditions call for chopped garlic to be covered in oil as a way to keep a ready supply of garlic at hand for cooking. When fresh garlic and oil are stored at room temperature, without the benefit of proper canning, the conditions are right for the growth of the botulinum bacteria which may already be on the garlic. Food made with infected garlic will cause botulism, a dangerous, often fatal, form of food poisoning.

A safe practice for keeping fresh garlic in oil is to make small amounts, store in the refrigerator and keep for only a week to ten days. Commercial products that list preservatives such as salt or acid (like vinegar) are safe to use but must be stored in the refrigerator once opened.

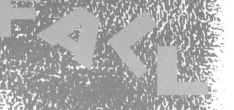

Ginseng Meusli

TIP

Use as a morning starter with milk or sprinkled over fruit or yogurt. It can also be used as a grain topping for fruit crisp and other desserts.

If fresh ginger root is not available, use 1/2 oz (15 g) dried whole ginger root simmered in water for 15 minutes, drained and minced. Reserve the liquid for tea.

Preheat oven to 375° F (190° C)
Large baking pan, lightly oiled

2 cups	spelt flakes	500 mL
1 cup	rolled oats	250 mL
1/2 cup	bran flakes	125 mL
1/2 cup	sunflower seeds	125 mL
2/3 cup	chopped almonds	150 mL
1/4 cup	chopped walnuts	50 mL
1/3 cup	sesame seeds	75 mL
1/2 cup	honey	125 mL
1/4 cup	grated ginseng	50 mL
2 tsp	ground cinnamon	10 mL
1 tsp	ground ginger	5 mL
1/2 cup	chopped dried apricots	125 mL
1/2 cup	raisins	125 mL

1. On prepared baking pan, spread spelt, oats, bran, sunflower seeds, almonds, walnuts and sesame seeds. Toast in preheated oven, stirring once, for 12 to 15 minutes or until lightly browned.

2. Meanwhile, in a small saucepan, heat honey, ginseng, cinnamon and ginger until just simmering. Remove from heat.

3. Remove grains from oven and transfer mixture to a large bowl. Drizzle with warm honey mixture. Add apricots and raisins; stir lightly to mix. Let cool and store in an airtight container.

Vegetable Frittata

Serves 4 to 6

TIP

Although traditionally served as a breakfast dish, the frittata is much more versatile. Cut into diamond shapes and top with herbed mayonnaise, smoked salmon or bean spread for hors d'oeuvres; cut into strips and serve as an accompaniment for soups or salads; or cut into larger squares and serve with pesto or red pepper sauce for an appetizer.

VARIATIONS

Substitute: Celery for leek; Green pepper for red pepper.

Add: 1 tsp (5 mL) cayenne pepper.

Preheat oven to 375° F (190° C)
9-inch (2.5 L) square baking dish, lightly oiled

2 cups	trimmed fresh spinach	500 mL
2 tbsp	butter	25 mL
1/2 cup	chopped onions	125 mL
2/3 cup	sliced leek, white and tender green parts only	150 mL
1/2 cup	chopped red bell peppers	125 mL
1/2 cup	shredded carrots	125 mL
6	large eggs	6
1/3 cup	milk	75 mL
1/4 cup	shredded Swiss cheese	50 mL
1/4 cup	shredded Cheddar cheese	50 mL
2 tsp	dried chopped oregano	10 mL
2 tsp	dried chopped sage	10 mL
2 tsp	dried chopped thyme	10 mL

1. Wash spinach and place wet leaves in a medium saucepan with lid. Turn heat to high and cook for about 2 minutes or until spinach is wilted. Remove from heat and drain. Allow spinach to cool; squeeze out excess moisture and chop.

2. Meanwhile, melt butter in a skillet over medium heat. Add onions, leek, peppers and carrots; cook until soft. Stir in spinach and distribute it evenly. Set aside to cool.

3. In a large bowl, beat eggs and milk together. Add Swiss cheese, Cheddar cheese, vegetable mixture, oregano, sage and thyme. Season to taste with salt and pepper. Pour into prepared baking dish. (Mixture can be prepared to this point and refrigerated several hours or overnight; return to room temperature before baking.)

4. Bake in preheated oven for 25 to 30 minutes or until lightly browned and set. Allow to cool for 10 minutes before cutting. Serve warm or at room temperature.

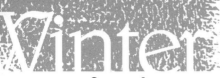

Vegetable Sushi with Wasabi-Mayonnaise Dip

TIP

Keep a bowl of vinegar water (1 cup [250 mL] warm water + 1 tsp [5 mL] vinegar) for dipping fingers and knife while making rolls.

VARIATIONS

Substitute: White vinegar for rice vinegar; White wine for sake; Any sprouts for broccoli sprouts.

Add: Sliced green or red pepper, avocado slices; Cooked crab or tuna in step 6.

2 cups	short-grain brown rice	500 mL
3 cups	water	750 mL
1/4 cup	rice vinegar	50 mL
2 tbsp	brown rice syrup	25 mL
2 tbsp	*sake*	25 mL
1/4 cup	toasted sesame seeds	50 mL
6	toasted *nori* sheets	6
1 cup	WASABI MAYONNAISE (see recipe, page 64)	250 mL
1	large zucchini, seeded, cut into 1/4-inch (5 mm) sticks and steamed 3 minutes or until just tender	1
1	large carrot, cut into 1/4-inch (5 mm) sticks and steamed 5 minutes or until just tender	1
1	small sweet potato, cut into 1/4-inch (5 mm) sticks and steamed 6 minutes or until just tender	1
1/2 cup	broccoli sprouts	125 mL

1. In a medium saucepan, combine rice and water; bring to a boil. Reduce heat, cover and simmer for 20 minutes or until water is absorbed and rice is tender but not mushy. Remove from heat; transfer to a large bowl.

2. Meanwhile, in a small saucepan, heat vinegar and brown rice syrup until syrup dissolves. Remove from heat and stir in *sake*. Set aside to cool.

3. Pour vinegar mixture over rice. Stir with a fork, making sure all grains are coated. Cover and allow rice to cool.

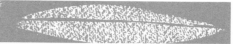

4. Place a sheet of waxed paper on a work surface and center one sheet of *nori*, shiny-side down and long side facing you, on top. Spread 1 cup (250 mL) of rice on nori, leaving a 1-inch (2.5 cm) border along top edge. Spread 1 tbsp (15 mL) WASABI MAYONNAISE over rice. Sprinkle with 2 tsp (10 mL) sesame seeds.

5. Lay 2 or 3 sticks of each vegetable in a horizontal line across center of *nori* sheet, letting them stick out slightly at ends. Top with one-sixth sprouts.

6. Moisten your fingers in vinegar water (see Tip, facing page) and roll evenly and tightly away from you, using waxed paper to help lift and roll. Rub vinegar water on edge of *nori* and press seam by rolling back and forth.

7. Dip a sharp knife into vinegar water and tip to coat whole blade. Trim ends; cut roll in half and each half into 3 equal pieces.

8. Repeat rolling-and-cutting procedure with remaining sheets of *nori* and filling.

9. On a serving platter, arrange sushi rolls. Serve immediately with extra WASABI MAYONNAISE, plain wasabi, pickled ginger and tamari sauce for dipping.

Winter

Wasabi-Mayonnaise

1 cup	mayonnaise	250 mL
2 tbsp	wasabi powder	25 mL

1. In a small bowl, whisk mayonnaise and wasabi together. Keep refrigerated for 1 to 2 days.

TIP

Wasabi is a light-green horseradish mustard that is very hot, the fumes of which can fill the nostrils as it is eaten. Start with tiny amounts to adjust to the degree of hotness. Wasabi is available in a paste or powder at Japanese markets or health/alternative stores. Use homemade mayonnaise (see recipe, page 177) or commercial soya mayonnaise.

VARIATIONS

Substitute: Dijon mustard for wasabi.

ROASTED SQUASH AND PEPPER SALAD (PAGE 88) ➤
OVERLEAF: AN ARRAY OF HEALING HERBS, OILS AND VINEGARS

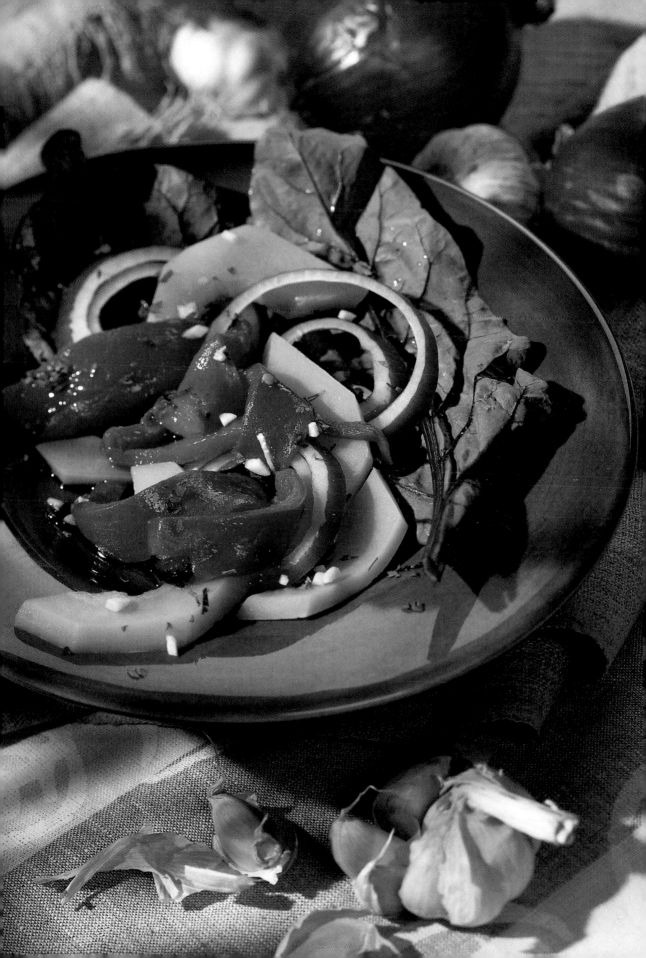

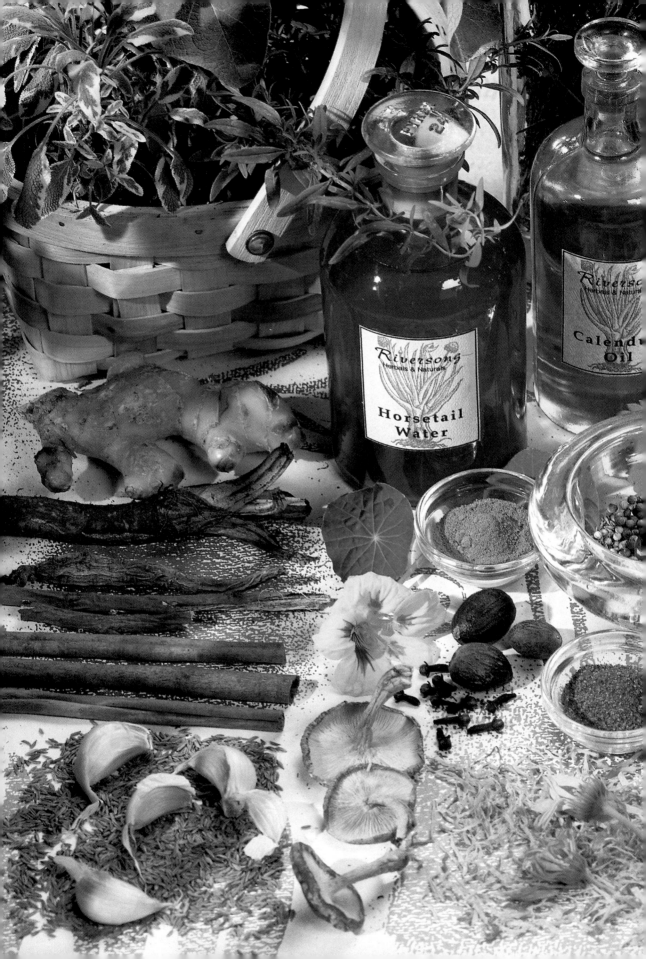

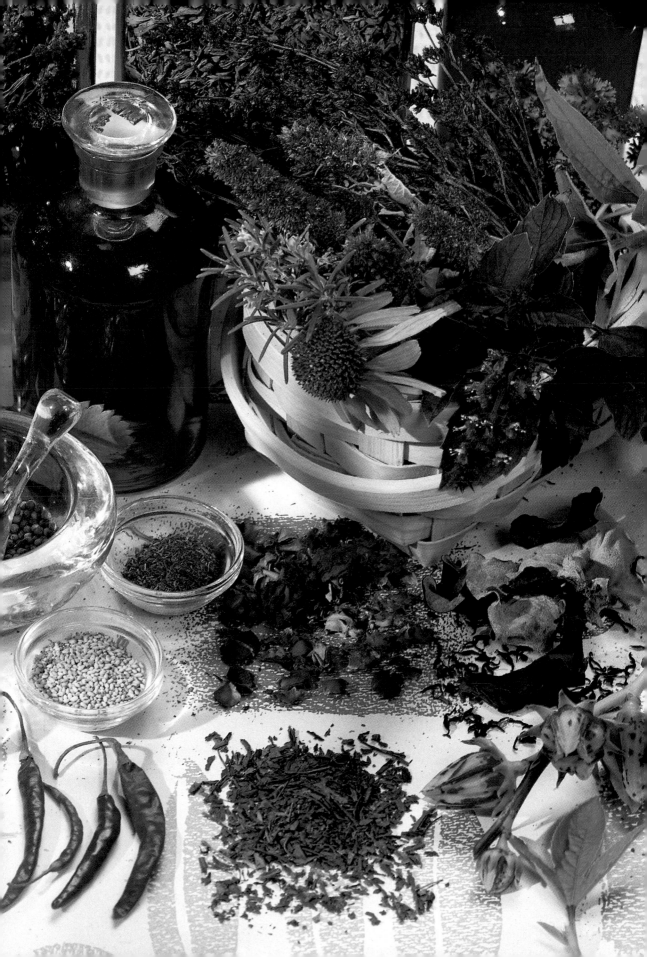

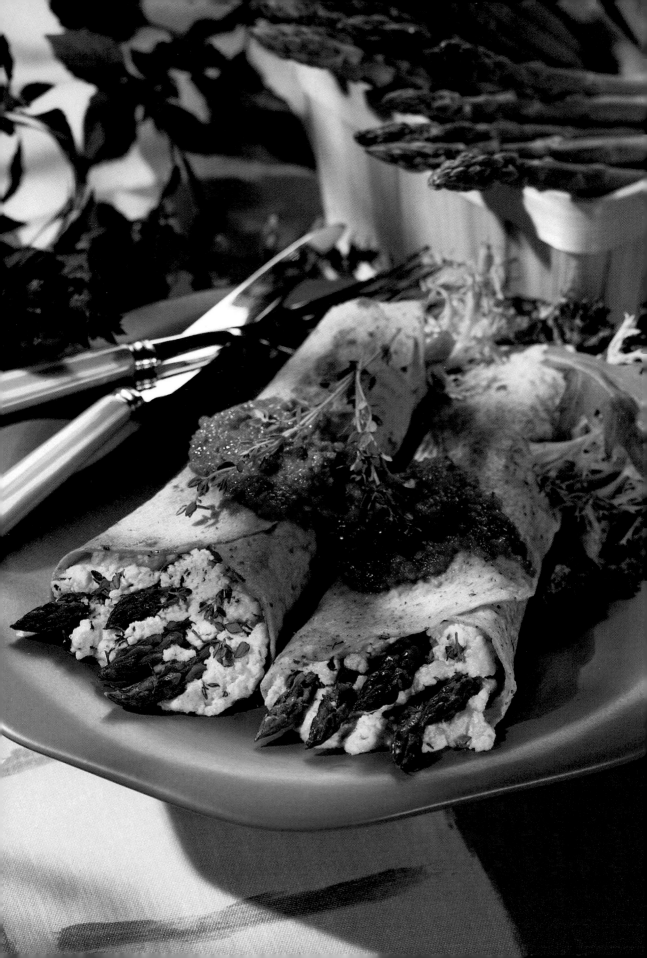

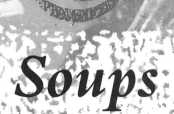

Soups

Cream of Mushroom Soup

Serves 4

TIP

Wild leeks are the first sign of the seasonal bounty nature offers — we wait all year for our brief, delicious encounter with them. They lure us out of housebound habits and contribute a light, fresh, clean flavor to any dish. Look for them in a deciduous wood near you (see facing page).

VARIATIONS

Substitute: 2 domestic leeks for wild leeks; Molasses or 1 tsp (5 mL) brown rice syrup for maple syrup; Regular mushrooms for shiitake or maitake mushrooms; Milk or 18% cream for soy milk.

Omit: Maple syrup if desired.

Add: 2 minced garlic cloves in step 1 if desired.

40	wild leeks	40
2 tbsp	butter	25 mL
1/2 cup	chopped onion	125 mL
1	domestic leek, white and tender green parts, chopped	1
2 cups	sliced shiitake or maitake mushrooms	500 mL
3 cups	stock	750 mL
1 tbsp	maple syrup	15 mL
2 cups	soy milk	500 mL

1. Clean wild leeks, separate white bulbs from leaves. Chop white bulb and purple stems. Slice green leaves and set aside.

2. In a large pot, heat butter over medium-low heat. Cook onion, wild leeks (except green leaves) and domestic leek, stirring often, for 25 minutes or until soft but not browned.

3. Add mushrooms to pot. Stir and cook for another 5 minutes, then add stock and maple syrup. If desired, season to taste with salt and pepper. Bring to a boil, reduce heat to simmer for at least 10 minutes or up to 1 hour. (Soup can be made up to 1 day ahead and stored in refrigerator. Bring back to simmer before continuing with step 4.)

4. Before serving, stir in sliced wild green leaves and soy milk. Heat through but do not boil. Serve immediately.

SOME WILD AND CULTIVATED HERBS FOR THE POT

Stinging Nettle (Urtica dioica)
Growing on waste ground, in ditches, against walls and fences, stinging nettle is well known for the bristly, stinging hairs that cover its leaves and stem. A familiar perennial, it grows from 3 to 6 feet (90 to 180 cm) high and has dull, dark green leaves similar to those of mint. Handle with gloves before cooking. Afterwards, you needn't worry, the sting disappears.

Marsh Marigold (Caltha palustris)
A low-growing, water-seeking plant that grows in a clump. Glossy, kidney-shaped leaves are light green and tender in spring and make good eating when stewed as greens. Yellow, buttercup-shaped flowers bloom from April to June.

Wild Leek (Allium tricoccum)
Often called "ramp", this onion-like plant has a white bulb that grows beneath the soil in low woods and thickets. It has one wide, flat, glossy green leaf and a definite garlic odor. One flower in an umbel forms, then the tops die back, making the bulbs almost impossible to find after spring.

Lovage (Levisticum officinale)
Rarely found in the wild, this perennial grows to 5 feet (150 cm). The leaves are glossy, dark green and similar in both appearance and smell to wild celery. Used in soups and stews, this fragrant herb was a popular ingredient of love potions during the Middle Ages.

Borage (Borago officinalis)
This hearty annual has erect stems and grows up to 2 feet (60 cm) high. The leaves are large, oval, alternate, deep green, covered with rough white hairs, and taste and smell like cucumbers. The blue star-shaped flowers are used in salads and drinks.

POT HERBS

The term "pot herb" comes from the early use of leaves (and sometimes roots) of plants in broths and soups. Before they were cultivated, many of our modern-day vegetables (such as cabbage, beet tops and lettuces) that were destined for the pot were gathered from hedgerows, fields and woods. All plants — large and small — were considered "herbs" if they served this function. While nourishing for soups and salads at any time, pot herbs were taken traditionally as spring cures to "cleanse" the blood after a heavy winter diet of salted meat and few fresh fruits and vegetables.

Spring Tonic Broth

**Makes about
12 cups (3 L)**

1	fresh burdock (root, stem and leaves)	1
2	fresh dandelions (roots, stems, leaves and flowers)	2
Quarter	green cabbage, cut into 4 pieces	Quarter
1	onion, quartered	1
1 cup	chopped wild leeks	250 mL
2	carrots, cut into chunks	2
2	apples, quartered	2
5	whole cloves	5
5	black peppercorns	5
5	allspice berries	5
3	dried astragalus root pieces	3
14 cups	water	3.5 L

1. Scrub roots and stems of all plants. Wash leaves, flowers, vegetables and fruit. Leave peel on vegetables and fruit if organic; do not core apples. Place all ingredients in a large stock pot.

2. Cover with water and bring to a boil, skimming off any foam that rises to the surface. Reduce heat, cover and simmer for at least 3 hours.

3. When ready to serve, strain off solids and discard. The broth will keep in a covered container in the refrigerator for up to 3 days or in the freezer for up to 3 months.

TIP

Spring, the season of Lent, has traditionally been a time for fasting. Spring herbs have therefore been valued for their role as natural digestion and liver stimulants. They gently nourish the liver and gall bladder, allowing the body to balance and renew itself after a winter of warmer, heavier foods. Even if you're not fasting, you'll enjoy the absence of fat and protein in this light and tasty broth. Be sure to keep the lid on during cooking to trap water-soluble nutrients in the steam.

VARIATIONS

Substitute: 1/2 cup (125 mL) dried burdock for fresh; 1/2 cup (125 mL) dried dandelion for fresh; Domestic leek for wild leeks; 1 tsp (5 mL) burdock and 1 tsp (5 mL) dandelion tincture for plants (added to finished broth).

Add: Parsnips, turnip, beet tops, mushrooms, or spinach, if desired; 1-inch (2.5 cm) piece dried ginseng root, if available.

Omit: Burdock, dandelion and astragalus if not available.

Spinach and Sea Vegetable Soup

Serves 6

Tip

A thick purée is the perfect foil for the slightly crisp, nutty-tasting strands of hijiki. Serve this robust soup with a salad and bread for a hearty spring lunch.

Variations

Substitute: One-quarter cabbage, coarsely chopped, for turnips; *Wakame* or *arame* for *hijiki*.

Add: 1/2 cup (125 mL) each chopped celery and green pepper in step 1 if desired.

3 tbsp	olive oil	45 mL
1 cup	chopped onions	250 mL
2	garlic cloves, finely chopped	2
2	carrots, chopped	2
1	leek, white and green tender part, chopped	1
2	turnips, chopped	2
7 cups	stock	1.75 L
10 oz	spinach, washed and trimmed	284 g
1 cup	*hijiki*	250 mL
2 tbsp	fresh chopped thyme	25 mL
1 tbsp	fresh chopped tarragon	15 mL

1. In a large pot, heat oil over medium heat. Add onions and sauté for 5 minutes or until soft. Stir in garlic, carrots, leek and turnips; cook for 5 minutes, stirring occassionally. Add 4 cups (1 L) stock; bring to a boil, reduce heat and simmer, covered, for 15 minutes or until vegetables are tender. Stir in spinach; cook for 2 minutes or until wilted. Remove from heat and allow to cool slightly.

2. In a food processor or blender, purée soup in batches, and return to pot. Add *hijiki*, thyme, tarragon and remaining stock. Simmer, covered, for 10 minutes or until *hijiki* is tender.

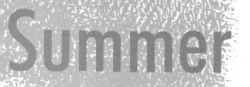

Hot-and-Sour Summer Soup

Serves 4

Tip

If you have the time in step 1, simmer this soup on low heat for 2 or 3 hours instead of 25 minutes. Keep the lid on in order to trap water-soluble nutrients that would otherwise escape in the steam.

Variations

Substitute: Burdock or dandelion for ginseng; Molasses or maple syrup for burdock syrup.

Add: 10 oz (284 g) package fresh spinach, coarsely chopped, in the last 3 minutes.

Omit: Ginseng if unavailable.

Soybeans and Menopause
Soybeans and soy products are high in phyto-estrogens (plant estrogens), which research has shown to help alleviate the symptoms of menopause. Phyto-estrogens in soybeans may also play a role in decreasing the risk of heart disease and cancer. Soy products contain isoflavones, which have effects similar to the female hormone estrogen and may play a role in reducing the risk of breast cancer in women.

Other foods high in phyto-estrogens are plums, carrots, apples, yams and coconuts.

Soup

2 tbsp	olive oil	30 mL
1 cup	chopped onions	250 mL
3 cups	diced turnips	750 mL
2	cloves garlic, minced	2
1 cup	sliced shiitake mushrooms	250 mL
1	piece dried ginseng root	1
5 cups	stock	1.25 L
3 tbsp	soya sauce	45 mL
3 tbsp	herbed vinegar	45 mL
1 tbsp	*burdock syrup* (see page 39 for technique)	15 mL
1/4 cup	fresh chopped parsley	50 mL
1/4 tsp	hot sauce	1 mL

Garnish

1	carrot, cut into matchsticks	1
8 oz	firm tofu, cut into 1/2-inch (1 cm) cubes	250 g
1/4 cup	chopped green onions	50 mL
1/4 cup	chopped fresh coriander	50 mL

1. In a large saucepan, heat oil over medium heat. Add onions and sauté for 5 minutes or until soft. Stir in turnip and garlic, cook another 5 minutes. Stir in mushrooms, ginseng, stock, soy sauce, vinegar, and syrup; cover and simmer for about 25 minutes or until vegetables are tender. Stir in parsley and hot sauce.

2. Remove ginseng root; chop fine and return to soup.

3. Divide garnish among 4 bowls; ladle hot soup over.

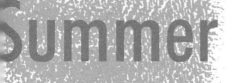
Mushroom-Almond Bisque

TIP

Designed to be a cold summer soup, this can also be served hot.

VARIATIONS

Omit: miso, if unavailable, adding more soya sauce to taste.

2 tbsp	olive oil	25 mL
1	leek, white and tender green part, sliced	1
20	shiitake *or* maitake mushrooms, sliced	20
1/4 cup	ground almonds	50 mL
2 cups	stock	500 mL
1	potato, cut into large chunks	1
2 tbsp	soya sauce	25 mL
2 tbsp	miso	25 mL
2 cups	soy milk	500 mL

1. In a large pot, heat oil over medium–low heat. Add leek and mushrooms; sauté for 10 minutes or until softened.

2. Stir in almonds, stock and potato; bring to a boil. Reduce heat and simmer, covered, for 15 minutes or until potatoes are tender. Allow to cool.

3. In a food processor or blender, purée mushroom mixture with soya sauce and miso until smooth. Stir in soy milk. Pour into a large soup tureen. Chill before serving.

MISO

Considered a key to the good health and longevity enjoyed by a majority of Asians, miso is a superb source of easily assimilated complete proteins, vitamins and minerals, including B12. Similar to other fermented foods like yogurt, unpasturized miso contains live microorganisms and enzymes that facilitate digestion.

Miso is made by combining cooked soybeans with salt and koji — a starter prepared by inoculating and incubating cooked rice or barley with beneficial mold spores. The mixture then ferments and the koji enzymes reduce proteins, starches and fats in the beans and grains to amino acids, simple sugars and fatty acids. The

flavor is distinct and mellow and the color darkens, depending on the amount of koji used and the length of fermentation. The texture is that of a thick paste.

Miso is used in soups, spreads, dips, sauces and gravy. It is available at Japanese markets and most alternative/health food stores.

Summer

Chilled Calendula-Strawberry Gazpacho

Serves 4 to 6

TIP

This is meant to be a chunky soup but may be completely puréed, if desired.

With its large, thin leaves, basil is easy to shred: remove stem and stack 3 or 4 fresh basil leaves; roll up from the wide end and slice into thin ribbons for garnish, salads, omelets or soups.

VARIATIONS

Substitute: Mixed berries (blueberries, raspberries, cherries) for strawberries; 2 tbsp (45 mL) calendula (or other edible petals) and 1 tbsp (15 mL) olive oil for calendula pesto; or any pesto for calendula pesto.

2 cups	chopped peeled tomatoes	500 mL
4 cups	sliced strawberries	1 L
3/4 cup	diced peeled seeded cucumber	175 mL
1/4 cup	shredded fresh basil	50 mL
3 tbsp	chopped fresh chives	45 mL
1 cup	apple juice	50 mL
1 cup	stock	50 mL
1/4 cup	raspberry vinegar	50 mL
3 tbsp	CALENDULA PESTO (see recipe, page 172)	45 mL

1. In a large bowl or soup tureen, combine all ingredients and mix well. In a food processor or blender, purée 3 cups (750 mL) of mixture. Combine with remaining mixture in bowl.

2. Cover bowl and refrigerate for at least 2 hours to chill and blend flavors. Season to taste with salt and pepper.

3. Serve cold, garnished with whole strawberries or calendula flowers.

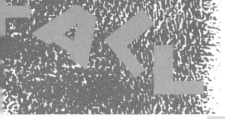

Corn and Rice Chowder with Parsley Persillade

Serves 4

TIP

Persillade is a fine mince of garlic and parsley added at the last to sautées, grilled dishes and casseroles, lentils, and vegetables (especially steamed peas and potatoes). Use it as a substitute for butter on vegetables.

VARIATIONS

Substitute: Regular milk for soy milk; Lentils or split peas for lima beans; Brown rice for wild rice.

2 tbsp	olive oil	25 mL
1 cup	chopped onions	250 mL
1 3/4 cup	sliced leeks, white and tender green parts only	425 mL
3 cups	soy milk	750 mL
1	can (14 oz [398 mL]) lima beans	1
1 1/3 cups	corn kernels	325 mL
1 cup	cooked wild rice	250 mL

Parsley Persillade

1/2 cup	finely chopped parsley	125 mL
1	clove garlic, minced	1
2 tbsp	finely chopped almonds	25 mL

1. In a large saucepan, heat oil over medium-low heat. Add onions and leeks; cook, stirring occasionally, for 20 minutes or until soft but not browned.

2. Meanwhile, in a small bowl, combine parsley, garlic and almonds. Set aside.

3. Stir milk and lima beans into onion mixture. In a blender or food processor, purée mixture in 2 batches and return to pot. Bring to a gentle simmer; stir in corn and rice. If desired, season to taste with salt. Cook over medium-low heat, covered and stirring occassionally, for 5 minutes or until corn is tender.

4. Serve immediately. Garnish with persillade.

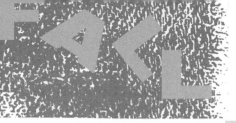

Curried Yam Soup

Serves 4

TIP

If canned coconut milk is unavailable, make your own. In a small bowl, combine 1/2 cup (125 mL) dessicated coconut and 1 3/4 cups (425 mL) hot milk. Allow to stand at least 1 hour. Strain and discard coconut before using the milk.

VARIATIONS

Substitute: Store-bought curry paste for home-made or 1 tbsp (15 mL) curry powder + 2 tsp (10 mL) turmeric; Any pesto for roasted garlic and red pepper pesto.

1 tbsp	olive oil	15 mL
1 cup	chopped onions	250 mL
1 tbsp	CURRY PASTE (see recipe, page 44)	15 mL
2	yams, peeled and diced	2
1 1/4 cups	chopped carrots	300 mL
3 cups	stock	750 mL
1/4 cup	chopped raisins	50 mL
1	can (14 oz [398 mL]) coconut milk	1
1/4 cup	ROASTED GARLIC AND RED PEPPER PESTO (see recipe, page 59), optional	50 mL

1. In a large saucepan, heat oil over medium heat. Add onion and curry paste; cook, stirring, for 4 minutes.

2. Stir in yams and carrots and cook for another 2 minutes. Stir in stock. Bring to a simmer and cook, covered, for 15 minutes. Add raisins and, if desired, season to taste with salt. Cook for 5 minutes or until vegetables are soft.

3. In two batches, using a blender or food processor, purée yam mixture. Return to pot, stir in coconut milk and heat through. To serve, ladle into soup bowls and float 1 tbsp (15 mL) roasted garlic and red pepper pesto on top.

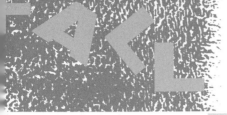

Roasted Vegetable and Tomato Bouillabaisse

Serves 4 to 6

TIP

Roasting is a dry-heat method of cooking vegetables that brings out the natural sugars in them.

To peel tomatoes, drop in boiling water for 5 to 10 seconds. Remove from water; core and peel.

VARIATIONS

Substitute: Any pesto for roasted garlic and red pepper pesto; One 28-oz (796 mL) can whole tomatoes for fresh tomatoes.

Preheat oven to 400° F (200° C)
Large baking pan, greased

1	onion, cut into 6 wedges	1
1	red bell pepper, cut into 1-inch (2.5 cm) pieces	1
3	carrots, cut into 1-inch (2.5 cm) pieces	3
2	parsnips, cut into 1-inch (2.5 cm) pieces	2
1	kohlrabi, coarsely chopped	1
1 tbsp	olive oil	15 mL
1/3 cup	ROASTED GARLIC AND RED PEPPER PESTO (see recipe, page 59)	75 mL
10 to 12	tomatoes, peeled and cut into wedges	10 to 12
1 cup	dulse	250 mL
1/4 cup	chopped fresh parsley	50 mL
4 to 6	fresh parsley sprigs	4 to 6

1. On prepared baking pan, combine onion, red pepper, carrots, parsnips and kohlrabi. Toss with oil and 1 tbsp (15 mL) water. If desired, season to taste with salt. Bake in preheated oven, stirring occasionally for 40 to 50 minutes or until vegetables are tender. Remove vegetables as they are done — some will cook faster than others.

2. In a large pot, combine roasted vegetables, pesto, tomatoes and dulse. Bring to a boil over medium-high heat; reduce heat and simmer, covered, for 20 minutes or until dulse and tomatoes are tender. Stir in parsley. Ladle into soup bowls and garnish each with a parsley sprig.

Winter

Sea Gumbo

Serves 4

TIP

The *arame* lends a taste of the sea to this dish. You can also add 1 lb (500 g) fresh shrimp or scallops in step 3 and simmer for 5 to 10 minutes. For a Louisiana style gumbo, add 1 tbsp (15 mL) Old Bay seasoning or 2 tsp (10 mL) cayenne pepper and a couple of drops of a hot sauce such as Tabasco.

VARIATIONS

Substitute: Zucchini for okra; 2 tbsp (30 mL) dried basil for fresh basil.

Omit: Basil, if unavailable.

3 tbsp	olive oil	45 mL
1 cup	chopped onions	250 mL
1 3/4 cups	sliced leeks, white and tender green parts	425 mL
3	cloves garlic, minced	3
1/2 cup	chopped celery stalk	125 mL
1/2 cup	chopped green pepper	125 mL
1/2 cup	chopped red bell pepper	125 mL
1	can (28 oz [796 mL]) tomatoes	1
1 cup	chopped okra	250 mL
1 cup	stock	250 mL
1	bay leaf	1
3 tbsp	chopped fresh thyme	45 mL
1 cup	*arame* or *hijiki*	250 mL
1/2 cup	shredded fresh basil	125 mL

1. In a large saucepan, heat oil over medium heat. Add onions and cook for 5 minutes or until soft. Add leeks and garlic; cook for 3 minutes. Add celery, green pepper and red pepper; cook another 5 minutes.

2. Stir in tomatoes, okra, stock, bay leaf, thyme and *arame*. If desired, season to taste with salt. Simmer, covered and stirring occassionally, for 35 minutes or until vegetables are tender. Stir in basil. Serve hot.

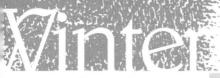

Cheddar Cheese and Root Soup

Serves 6

TIP

This soup can simmer all day before the cheese and milk are added. Just keep an eye on the liquid and add more when required.

VARIATIONS

Substitute: Regular milk for soy milk.

Omit: Ginseng if unavailable.

3 tbsp	olive oil	45 mL
1 3/4 cups	chopped leeks, white and tender green parts	425 mL
1 cup	chopped onions	250 mL
2	cloves garlic, minced	2
1 1/4 cups	chopped parsnips	300 mL
1 1/4 cups	chopped carrots	300 mL
1 cup	chopped potatoes	250 mL
1 cup	chopped rutabaga	250 mL
1 tbsp	dried thyme	15 mL
1 tbsp	dried sage	15 mL
2 cups	stock	500 mL
1	piece dried ginseng root	1
2 cups	soy milk	500 mL
2 cups	shredded Cheddar cheese	500 mL

1. In a large pot, heat oil over medium heat. Add leeks, onions, garlic, parsnips, carrots, potatoes, rutabaga, thyme and sage; cook for 10 minutes, stirring often.

2. Add stock and ginseng. If desired, season to taste with salt and pepper. Bring to a boil; reduce heat and simmer, covered, for 15 to 20 minutes or until vegetables are tender.

3. Remove ginseng; chop fine and return to pot.

4. With a slotted spoon, remove about 1/2 cup (125 mL) vegetables to a bowl; mash with a fork or potato masher. Return to pot. Add milk. Heat through but do not allow to boil. Stir in cheese until melted. Serve immediately.

Roasted Squash, Caramelized Onion and Garlic Soup

Serves 8 to 10

TIP

Be sure to make two batches, freezing one, of this exquisite soup — it will transport you to a fine French bistro on the Mediterranean.

VARIATIONS

Substitute: Turban for butternut squash; Yellow onions for red.

SERVING SUGGESTIONS

Ladle soup into large, flameproof soup bowls and float two rounds of soft goat's cheese in the center. Place under broiler for 1 to 2 minutes or until cheese melts slightly. Garnish with fresh rosemary sprig. Serve immediately.

Ladle into soup bowls and grate Cheddar or Swiss cheese into center; or simply garnish with fresh sprigs of rosemary or marjoram.

For an extra-rich soup, stir in 1 cup (250 mL) 18% cream into soup, heat through and serve immediately.

Preheat oven to 400° F (200° C)
Large baking pan, greased
Small baking pan

1	large butternut squash	1
3	large red onions, peeled and cut into eighths	3
12	cloves garlic, peeled	12
3 tbsp	olive oil	45 mL
2 tbsp	dried rosemary	25 mL
2 tbsp	dried thyme	25 mL
4 1/2 to 6 cups	stock	1.125 to 1.5 L
2 tbsp	balsamic vinegar	25 mL
1 tbsp	molasses	15 mL

1. Prick squash and place on small baking pan. Bake in preheated oven for 70 minutes, turning once, until tender. Remove from oven; allow to cool.

2. In a large bowl, toss onions with oil. If desired, season to taste with salt. Place on large baking pan with squash; bake for 20 minutes. Add garlic to pan; stir to coat well. Bake, stirring occassionally, for another 30 minutes or until onions are very soft and golden brown. Remove from oven; allow to cool slightly.

3. Meanwhile, cut squash in half, lengthwise. Remove and discard seeds; scoop out flesh. In batches in a food processor, with about 1/2 cup (125 mL) stock per batch, process squash, caramelized onion mixture, rosemary, thyme and vinegar until smooth. (At this point, mixture can be refrigerated or frozen in 2-cup [500 mL] portions.)

4. When ready to serve, place purée in a large soup pot. Stir in remaining stock until desired consistency is achieved. Blend well and heat through.

Onions (Allium)

There is in every
cook's opinion
No savoury dish
without an onion
But less your kissing
should be spoiled
The onion must be
thoroughly boiled.

Jonathan Swift
Gulliver's Travels

There are an estimated 500 to 600 species in the Allium genus, including leeks, chives and garlic, and most are native to the Northern Hemisphere. In ancient times, onions were known as an aphrodisiac, the Egyptians regarding it as a sign of vitality. All contain sulfur compounds that convert to different sulfides, flavonoids, coumarin and ellagic acid — all of which account for their medicinal qualities and their different flavors.

Actions: *anti-cancer, antioxidant, circulatory and digestive stimulant, antiseptic, detoxifying, lowers cholesterol, hypotensive, hypoglycemic, diuretic.*

Uses: *In traditional folk medicine, people have used onions as a blood purifier. Research shows that onions help prevent thrombosis, reduce high blood pressure, lower blood sugar, prevent inflammatory responses, and they may inhibit the growth of cancer cells. Shallots, yellow and red onions (not white onions) are the richest dietary source of quercetin, a potent antioxidant and cancer-inhibiting phytochemical.*

Some Types of Onions:

Bermuda: *A small-to medium-sized white onion with a sharp, hot flavor; good for stews and sautés.*

Egyptian: *An ornamental onion with small, edible bulbs that appear on the top of the flower stalks. If left uncut, the onions gradually increase in size until they become heavy enough to arch over and root in the ground. The green, flat, hollow leaves are used for stir-fries and salads, or any recipe where chives are used; the tiny, aerial onions are used whole, as you would pearl onions.*

Maui: *Grown in Hawaii, available April through June, the Maui onion is a "fresh" or seasonal variety of onion. Sweet tasting, mild and juicy, it is stuffed and roasted, stir-fried and used in onion soup.*

Pearl: *A small, mature bulb about 1 1/4 inches (3.5 cm) in diameter, usually white but can be yellow. When cooked or blanched, pearl onions have a sweet flavor. Their size lends them for use whole, on kebabs, creamed or gratinéed, in pickles, stews and soups, and as a garnish for drinks and salads.*

Red: *Also called Italian red onions, these large, reddish-purple onions are flat on both ends. Their mild flavor makes them perfect for slicing and using raw in sandwiches, wraps, burgers and salads.*

Scallions: *Also called spring or green onions, the white bulb and green, flat, hollow leaves are both used. Mild in taste, they are served whole, raw as a garnish for sandwiches or salads, and are chopped and included in salads, stir-fried vegetables, and with light pasta sauces.*

Shallots: *These brown, small onions are tear-drop shaped and mild tasting. They are close relatives to garlic because they separate into cloves. Shallots are used often in French sauces and ragouts.*

Spanish: *Also called yellow onions, this variety is the most commonly used. Its crisp, sweet flesh can be used in any recipe. The peak time for Spanish onions is September and October.*

Vidalia: *A large, flat-topped onion with dull, gold-colored skin and pale, crisp, white flesh. It is available June through August. A granex hybrid that is ideally suited to the soil and climate in and around Georgia, the sugar content of this variety is higher than that of apples, which makes them an excellent choice for eating raw or for recipes that require caramelizing.*

Winter

Creamy Tomato-Thyme Soup

Serves 4

TIP

If you use a food processor to purée this soup, it will contain some fine bits. Using a blender will liquify the mixture, leaving it smoother.

VARIATIONS

Substitute: 2 carrots or parsnips *or* 1 apple for kohlrabi.

Add: 1 tsp (5 mL) grated nutmeg and garlic cloves; for a creamier soup, 1/2 cup (125 mL) 18% cream in last 5 minutes before puréeing.

1 tbsp	olive oil	15 mL
1 cup	finely chopped onions	250 mL
2	cloves garlic, minced	2
1 cup	finely chopped kohlrabi	250 mL
1 cup	shredded rutabaga	250 mL
1	can (28 oz [796 mL]) tomatoes	1
1 cup	stock	250 mL
2 tbsp	dried thyme	25 mL
2 tbsp	molasses	25 mL
1 tbsp	apple cider vinegar	15 mL

1. In a large pot, heat oil over medium heat. Add onions; cook for 5 minutes. Stir in garlic, kohlrabi and rutabaga; cook for another 3 minutes.

2. Add tomatoes, stock, thyme, molasses and vinegar. If desired, season to taste with salt and pepper. Bring to a boil; reduce heat and simmer, covered, for 45 to 50 minutes or until vegetables are soft.

3. Purée soup in batches in a blender or food processor. (Soup can be prepared up to 1 day in advance and refrigerated.) Heat through before serving.

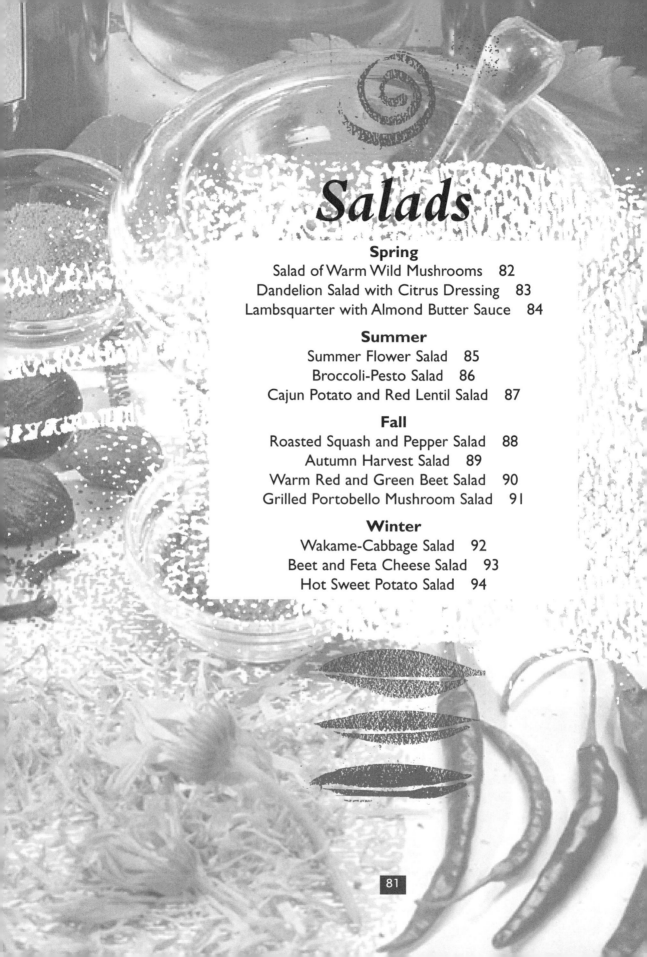

Salads

Spring
Salad of Warm Wild Mushrooms   82
Dandelion Salad with Citrus Dressing   83
Lambsquarter with Almond Butter Sauce   84

Summer
Summer Flower Salad   85
Broccoli-Pesto Salad   86
Cajun Potato and Red Lentil Salad   87

Fall
Roasted Squash and Pepper Salad   88
Autumn Harvest Salad   89
Warm Red and Green Beet Salad   90
Grilled Portobello Mushroom Salad   91

Winter
Wakame-Cabbage Salad   92
Beet and Feta Cheese Salad   93
Hot Sweet Potato Salad   94

Salad of Warm Wild Mushrooms

Serves 4

In North America, the term "mesclun" is applied to any mixture of tender young lettuces, herbs and other greens. It originated in France where it is a combination of chervil, arugula, lettuce and endive in precise proportions. In North America the ingredients are often organic and may include a variety of greens and herbs. Some mesclun mixtures also include edible flowers.

Some of the greens in mesclun are not new. In the 16th and 17th centuries, "sallet" was the only vegetable mentioned and would have contained 20 or 30 ingredients and at least a dozen greens. Mâche, dandelion, watercress, miner's lettuce, mustard greens, arugula, spinach, marsh marigold, and purslane were well known to cooks at that time.

Preheat oven to 375° F (190° C)
Baking sheet, lightly oiled

8 oz	wild mushrooms such as chanterelles, ceps, or oyster mushrooms, cleaned and sliced	250 g
1/4 cup	olive oil	50 mL
2 tbsp	chopped fresh chives	5 mL
1	large clove garlic, chopped	1
4 oz	soft goat cheese, cut into 4 rounds	125 g
4 cups	mesclun *or* french sorrel	1 L
2 tbsp	chopped fresh hyssop *or* sage	25 mL
2 tbsp	fresh tarragon	25 mL
2 tbsp	fresh chervil	25 mL
1/2 cup	fresh nasturtium flowers	125 mL
2 tbsp	fresh chive flowers	25 mL
2 tbsp	balsamic vinegar	25 mL

1. In a skillet over medium heat, heat 2 tbsp (25 mL) oil. Add chives and garlic; cook for 1 to 2 minutes. Add mushrooms and sauté for 1 minute or until barely tender. Season to taste with salt and pepper. Using a slotted spoon, lift mushrooms out of pan onto prepared baking sheet, dividing into 4 portions. Place goat cheese in center of each portion. Bake in preheated oven for about 4 minutes, allowing cheese to melt but not brown.

2. Meanwhile, wash and dry mesclun, hyssop and tarragon. Place in a medium bowl and toss with nasturtium and chive flowers. Divide into 4 portions and arrange on plates.

3. Add remaining oil to skillet over medium heat. Stir to collect pan juices and bits. Add vinegar; simmer until slightly reduced.

4. Spoon hot mushrooms and their juices over mesclun mixture; drizzle with hot oil and vinegar. Serve immediately.

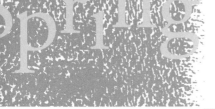

Dandelion Salad with Citrus Dressing

TIP

The light citrus dressing is just right to allow the tangy, bitter taste of the dandelion leaves to have their effect on the body. Should you choose not to let the bitter quality predominate, add 1/2 cup (125 mL) each of chopped apricots and raisins and 1/4 cup (50 mL) almond slivers.

VARIATIONS

Substitute: Arugula, mizuna, mesclun or sorrel for dandelion leaves; Half red onion, thinly sliced, for wild leeks; Fresh rose petals or nasturtium flowers for dandelion petals.

Omit: Dandelion petals if unavailable.

1/2 cup	fresh orange juice	125 mL
2 tbsp	fresh lemon juice	25 mL
2 tbsp	chopped fresh lemon thyme	25 mL
2 tbsp	chopped fresh lemon balm	25 mL
2/3 cup	extra virgin olive oil	150 mL
2 cups	fresh dandelion leaves, washed and patted dry	500 mL
2 cups	fresh spinach, washed and patted dry	500 mL
1 cup	sliced wild leeks	250 mL
1/2 cup	alfalfa sprouts	125 mL
1/4 cup	finely minced fresh parsley	50 mL
1/4 cup	fresh dandelion petals	50 mL

1. In a clean jar with a tight-fitting lid or a mixing bowl, combine orange juice, lemon juice, lemon thyme, lemon balm and olive oil. Shake or whisk well to combine. If desired, season to taste with salt.

2. In a large salad bowl, combine dandelion leaves, spinach, leeks, alfalfa sprouts, parsley and dandelion petals. Drizzle with enough dressing to coat leaves and toss well.

IN PRAISE OF BITTERNESS

Herbalists champion the bitter taste of some herbs that North Americans have, until recently, shunned. It is generally agreed that bitters support the heart, small intestines and liver, as well as reduce fever. As one of the four tastes — sweet, salty, bitter and sour — bitter is just beginning to take its rightful place in meals. The astringent taste of greens such as endive, chicory, sheep sorrel, radicchio, dandelion and yellow dock awakens the palate and poises it for more balanced tastes. The digestive tonic action promotes the secretion of hydrochloric acid which aids digestion. A small, light salad of bitter greens is an excellent tool for whetting the appetite.

Scientists say we have about 10,000 taste buds, with each one lasting not much longer than a week before it is shed and regenerated. Taste buds are clusters of cells on the tongue and in the mouth that relay the four tastes to the brain. Some herbalists and ancient traditions link the four tastes to mental effects on the body. For example, a balanced intake of bitter flavors could be thought to encourage honesty, integrity, optimism and a loving heart.

Lambsquarter with Almond Butter Sauce

Serves 4

TIP

Make the sauce first so that it is ready when the greens are.

This sauce is thinner than most nut-butter sauces so as not to over-power the delicate texture of the cooked greens. Add more water or stock if the sauce is too thick to mix with the greens.

Use natural, raw almonds with the skin still intact.

If using kale to replace lambsquarter greens, remove the tough central stem first.

VARIATIONS

Substitute: Peanut butter or cashew butter for almond butter; Mustard, beet or turnip greens, spinach, cress, kale or French sorrel for lamb-squarter greens; Dried apricots for raisins.

Add: 1 cup (250 mL) chopped dandelion or burdock root in step 1; 1 cup (250 mL) sliced mushrooms with onions in step 2.

1/2 cup	almond butter	125 mL
1/4 cup	lemon juice	50 mL
2 tbsp	soya sauce	25 mL
1/3 cup	warm water (or as needed)	75 mL
8 cups	water	2 L
6 cups	lambsquarter greens, washed	1.5 L
2 tbsp	olive oil	25 mL
2	cloves garlic, minced	2
1	onion, chopped	1
1/4 cup	chopped raisins	50 mL
1/4 cup	chopped unblanched almonds	50 mL

1. In a small mixing bowl, combine almond butter, lemon juice and soya sauce. Gradually stir in warm water until sauce reaches a creamy consistency.

2. In a large pot over medium–high heat, bring water to a boil. Add greens; cook uncovered for 2 to 3 minutes. Drain and rinse with cold water, press out excess liquid and chop coarsely.

3. In a medium-sized skillet, heat oil over medium heat. Add garlic and onion; cook for 5 minutes or until soft. Stir in greens; cook, stirring, for 2 minutes or until tender.

4. Toss cooked greens with 1/2 cup (125 mL) sauce, raisins and almonds.

Summer Flower Salad

Serves 4

TIP

Use the flowering tops of any herbs (mint, sage, thyme, hyssop); the petals of pinks, calendula, echinacea, elecampane; or elderflowers, nasturtums and violets for this dramatic, simple salad. Mix herb leaves from hyssop, nasturtium, savory or thyme in with the greens.

VARIATIONS

Substitute: Any sprouts for sunflower sprouts; Pecans or walnuts for almonds.
Add: 1/2 cup (125 mL) sliced strawberries, raspberries, blueberries or cherries.

3 cups	torn mixed greens such as mizuna, rocket, watercress, alfalfa	750 mL
1/2 cup	sunflower sprouts	125 mL
2 tbsp	chopped raisins	25 mL
2 tbsp	chopped apricots	25 mL
2 tbsp	chopped almonds	25 mL
1/4 cup	olive oil	50 mL
2 tbsp	raspberry vinegar *or* strawberry vinegar	25 mL
2 cups	flowers (see list below)	500 mL

1. In a large bowl, combine greens, sprouts, raisins, apricots and almonds.

2. In a jar with a tight-fitting lid, combine oil and vinegar. If desired, season to taste with salt and pepper. Shake well and toss with salad.

3. Arrange salad on a large serving platter. Top with flowers.

EDIBLE FLOWERS

Most flowers from culinary or medicinal herbs are edible. Be sure that flowers and herbs are grown pesticide-free and that you do not wildcraft at the sides of busy roads. Add any of the following petals or whole flowers to summer salads or use as a colorful garnish:

Bergamot	*Lavender*	
Borage	*Day lilies*	
Calendula	*Nasturtium*	
Chicory	*Pansy*	
Chives	*Rose*	
Clove pinks	*Rosemary*	
Dandelion	*Sage*	
Hollyhock	*Thyme*	
Hyssop		

Broccoli-Pesto Salad

3/4 cup	fresh basil pesto	175 mL
3 tbsp	balsamic vinegar	45 mL
2	bunches fresh broccoli, parboiled and chopped	2
1 cup	broccoli sprouts	250 mL
2 cups	cooked whole wheat pasta	500 mL

1. In a large salad bowl, whisk together pesto and vinegar.

2. Add broccoli, sprouts and pasta. Toss to mix well. Serve at room temperature.

TIP

Parboil broccoli by immersing in a large pot of boiling water, uncovered, for 2 to 3 minutes. Drain and cool in a colander.

This salad is quite attractive served in a white dish using spiral-shaped pasta.

VARIATIONS

Substitute: Cauliflower flowerettes for broccoli; Any other pesto for basil pesto.

Add: 1/2 cup (125 mL) chopped nuts; Half red onion, thinly sliced.

POTATOES (SOLANUM TUBEROSUM)

The poisonous properties of potato stalks and leaves are not found in the tubers of the potato plant because they grow underground and are not touched by light. However, when potatoes are exposed to daylight, they will turn green and begin to develop the same poisonous properties as the stalks and leaves.

Native to the Americas, potatoes were introduced to Europe in the 16th century. Raw potatoes were carried in pockets or pouches as protection against rheumatism and gout. A poultice of raw pounded potato was applied to burns and scalds.

The high starch content makes potato fermentation easy for alcohol production. Potato juice has been used to aid digestive disorders such as indigestion, colic, gastritis and ulcers.

White potatoes contain anti-cancer properties and are high in potassium, which may help prevent high blood pressure and strokes. Low in fat and a good source of carbohydrate, B vitamins, vitamin C and minerals when baked or steamed in its skin, the potato is easily digested and delivers nutrients to the body.

Actions: antioxidant, antiviral, anti-inflammatory, digestive.

Summer

Cajun Potato and Red Lentil Salad

Serves 4

TIP

Double the amounts for a summer picnic or barbecue.

If not accustomed to cayenne pepper, start with 1/4 tsp (1 mL) and gradually add more to taste.

Large sprouts such as broccoli or sunflower work well in this recipe, but you can use any type available.

VARIATIONS

Substitute: Green onions for scapes; Sour cream for yogurt; More or less cayenne pepper, to taste.

1/2 cup	red lentils, rinsed	125 mL
1 1/2 cups	water	375 mL
4	large potatoes, scrubbed and halved	4
1/3 cup	flaxseed oil	75 mL
3 tbsp	raspberry vinegar	45 mL
2 tbsp	sesame seeds	25 mL
2 tbsp	poppy seeds	25 mL
2 tbsp	flax seeds	25 mL
1/3 cup	plain yogurt	75 mL
1 tsp	cayenne powder	5 mL
1/4 cup	chopped scapes	50 mL
3	hardboiled eggs, cut into wedges	3
1/4 cup	large sprouts (see Tip, at left)	50 mL

1. In a saucepan combine lentils with water. Bring to a boil; reduce heat and simmer gently for 20 minutes or until lentils are tender. Allow to cool in a colander.

2. Meanwhile, in a medium saucepan, cover potatoes with cold water. Bring to a boil, reduce heat and simmer for 20 to 25 minutes or until just tender. Drain and rinse with cold water. When cool enough to handle, cut into 1-inch (2.5 cm) pieces.

3. In a small bowl, whisk together oil, raspberry vinegar, sesame seeds, poppy seeds, flax seeds, yogurt and cayenne. Season to taste with salt and pepper.

4. In a large salad bowl, combine cooled lentils, potatoes and scapes. Gently stir in dressing. Garnish with egg wedges and sprouts.

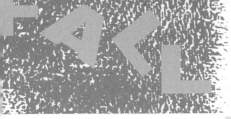

Roasted Squash and Pepper Salad

Serves 6

TIP

Easy to make, this simple salad or side dish can be made in advance.

	Preheat oven to 400° F (200° C) Baking dish	
1	small butternut, acorn or buttercup squash	1
1/2 cup	thinly sliced red onions	125 mL
2 cups	ROASTED RED PEPPERS IN MARINADE (see recipe, page 58)	500 mL

1. Prick squash in several places with a knife and place in baking dish. Bake in preheated oven for 45 minutes or until tender when pierced with a sharp knife. Remove from oven and allow to cool.

2. Cut squash in half lengthwise. Scoop out seeds; cut peel away from flesh. Cut each half lengthwise into 3 slices. Arrange squash slices on 6 plates alternately with onion slices. Spoon roasted red peppers over top, allowing marinade to drizzle over squash and onions. Serve at room temperature.

ROASTING AND CARAMELIZING VEGETABLES

Roasting fruit or vegetables is a technique that requires a higher heat than baking. This fast cooking method seals in the vegetables' juices and caramelizes the natural sugars on the outside, concentrating and deepening the flavors. Thick, firm and juicy-fleshed fruit like plums, apricots and cherries, and all manner of vegetables — such as beets, onions, squash, turnip, carrots, parsnips, eggplant, sweet potatoes, corn on the cob and asparagus are all excellent when roasted.

TO ROAST VEGETABLES: On a baking sheet, spread trimmed and quartered or coarsely chopped vegetables in a single layer. Drizzle with 1 to 2 tbsp (15 to 25 mL) olive oil and roast at 400° F (200° C) in the lower half of the oven (to maximize caramelization of the natural sugars) for 25 to 45 minutes. Roasted fruit and vegetables will blacken slightly around the edges and will be shrivelled in appearance. For this reason, they are often used in soups and puréed dishes.

TO ROAST GARLIC BUDS: In dishes where a more mellow garlic flavor is desired, whole head of garlic is roasted and used. Slice the tips off the top of the cloves and set, cut side up, on a baking sheet. Drizzle with 1 tsp (5 mL) olive oil and roast at 400° F (200° C) for 35 to 40 minutes, until cloves are very soft.

Note: If using a clay roaster with a lid, roast at 375° F (190° C) for 30 to 35 minutes.

Autumn Harvest Salad

TIP

Carrots, turnip and beets can be cut into julienne strips for this recipe. For carrots, cut into 2-inch (5 cm) lengths, then slice each length in 1/4-inch (1 cm) slices. Stack the slices and cut 1/4-inch (1 cm) sticks. For turnips, cut 1/4-inch (1 cm) slices. Stack and cut 1/4-inch (1 cm) sticks.

For fresh thyme, use the leaves only, stripping them away from the tough stem.

VARIATIONS

Substitute: Any sprout for bean sprouts; Any nuts for almonds.

1 cup	shredded carrots	250 mL
1/2 cup	shredded turnips	125 mL
1/2 cup	shredded beets	125 mL
1	apple, diced	1
1 cup	bean sprouts	250 mL
2	green onions, chopped	2
1 tbsp	fresh thyme leaves	15 mL
1 tbsp	chopped fresh sage	15 mL
1/4 cup	olive oil	50 mL
2 tbsp	soya sauce	25 mL
2 tbsp	lemon juice	25 mL
1 tbsp	minced candied ginger	5 mL
1 tsp	sesame oil	5 mL
1	clove garlic, minced	1
1/4 cup	coarsely chopped almonds	50 mL

1. In a large salad bowl, combine carrots, turnips, beets, apple, bean sprouts, green onions, thyme and sage.

2. In a small bowl or jar with a tight-fitting lid, combine olive oil, soya sauce, lemon juice, candied ginger, sesame oil and garlic. Whisk or shake until well mixed. Drizzle over salad; toss to mix well. Garnish with almonds.

Warm Sweet-and-Sour Beet Salad

Serves 4 to 6

TIP

This salad can also be served cold the next day.

Remember to peel non-organic fruits and vegetables.

VARIATIONS

Substitute: Apple cider for apple juice; 4 cups (1 L) washed torn spinach for beet tops; Red wine vinegar for raspberry vinegar.

4	beets, including greens	4
2 tbsp	olive oil	25 mL
1	red onion, quartered	1
1/2 cup	stock	125 mL
1/2 cup	apple juice	125 mL
2	green apples, cored and quartered	2
10 to 12	dried apricots, quartered	10 to 12
2 tbsp	raspberry vinegar	25 mL

1. Cut greens off beets; wash thoroughly. Chop stems and shred tender leaves; set aside. Trim root and coarse skin off beets; cut into wedges.

2. In a Dutch oven or roasting pan with lid, heat oil over medium heat. Add onion and cook for 5 minutes or until tender. Add beets, stock and apple juice. Bring to a boil; cover, reduce heat and simmer for about 20 minutes.

3. Stir in apples; cover and cook, stirring occasionally, for 6 minutes or until beets are tender. Stir in apricots, vinegar and beet stems and tops. Increase heat to medium-high; cook, stirring, for 10 minutes or until liquid evaporates and vegetabes are coated with sauce. Season to taste with salt and pepper if desired. Serve warm.

BEETS

Beets have a long history of use in Europe. In the 16th century, referring to beet tops as "beet," herbalist John Gerard wrote: "The greater red Beet or Roman Beet, boyled and eaten with oyle, vinegre and pepper, is a most excellent and delicat sallad: but what might be made of the red and beautifull root...I refer unto the curious and cunning cooke, who no doubt when hee had the view thereof, and is assured that it is both good and wholesome, will make thereof many and divers dishes, both faire and good."

Cooking tips: Organic beets are dense with a better texture than non-organic. Always leave the skin on when steaming, roasting or boiling beets. The skin will slip off easily when cool enough to handle and vitamin and mineral loss is minimal with this method.

To roast beets: Scrub beets, cut off ends, place on a baking sheet and cover with an ovenproof bowl. Bake at 400° F (200° C) for about 1 hour. Remove skins; slice, dice or serve whole. Serve as you would baked potatoes, with sour cream, yogurt, butter or olive oil.

Continued on facing page...

Grilled Portobello Mushroom Salad

Serves 4

TIP

Mushrooms are easy to grill on the barbecue.
Garnish with fresh sage sprigs.

VARIATIONS

Substitute: Melted butter for olive oil; Apple juice for orange juice; Apples for pears; Feta cheese for blue cheese.

	Preheat broiler or start barbecue	
4	large portobello mushrooms, washed	4
4 tbsp	olive oil	50 mL
1 cup	chopped onions	250 mL
2 tbsp	chopped fresh sage	25 mL
2/3 cup	orange juice	150 mL
4	pears, cored, halved and cut into thin strips	4
1/4 cup	crumbled blue cheese	50 mL

1. Remove stems from mushrooms and chop if not too woody; set aside. Brush caps with 2 tbsp (25 mL) oil. Arrange on a baking sheet or barbecue grill. Place on top rack in oven and broil or grill for 3 minutes per side or until lightly browned. Remove from oven and cut into thin strips.

2. In a large skillet, heat remaining 2 tbsp (25 mL) oil over medium heat. Add onions and chopped mushroom stems; cook for 8 minutes or until very soft. Add sage and orange juice; increase heat to medium-high and boil for 2 to 3 minutes or until juice thickens and is reduced by about one-half. Stir in mushroom strips. Season to taste with salt and pepper if desired.

3. In a large bowl, gently toss pears with mushroom mixture. Sprinkle cheese over top. Serve warm.

Actions: tonic.

Uses: The yang energy of beets is grounding and warming and that makes them a perfect food for winter. Rich in beta carotene and high in the enzyme betaine (which nourishes and strengthens the liver and gall bladder), beets are also an excellent source of potassium. With 8% chlorine, beets are also a good bet as liver, kidney and gall bladder cleansers. In fact, raw beet juice taken several times a day is recommended for weak or diseased kidneys. The stimulating effect of chlorine on the lymph system makes them a good all-round vegetable for the diet.

Food Value:
(per 100 g beet root)
1 g fiber
16 mg calcium
60 mg sodium
335 mg potassium
10 mg vitamin C
20 IU vitamin A
0.7 mg iron

(per 100 g beet greens)
1.3 g fiber
119 mg calcium
3.3 mg iron
130 mg sodium
570 mg potassium
6,100 IU vitamin A
30 mg vitamin C

Winter

Wakame-Cabbage Salad

TIP

Either *arame*, dulse, *hijiki* or *wakame* may be used in this recipe. Look for sea herbs at your local alternative/health food store and some super-markets.

VARIATIONS

Substitute: 2/3 cup (150 mL) freshly made mayonnaise (see page 177) for dressing.

Add: Chopped broccoli, cauliflower, shredded turnip, rutabaga, or bean sprouts.

Carrots

Actions: antioxidant, anti-cancer, artery-protecting, expectorant, antiseptic, diuretic, immune-boosting

Uses: Carrots are extremely nutritious and rich in vitamins A, B and C, iron, calcium, potassium and sodium. They have a cleansing effect on the liver and digestive system, help counter the formation of kidney stones and relieve arthritis and gout. Their antioxidant properties from carotenoids (including beta-carotene) have been shown to cut cancer risk, protect against arterial and heart disease and lower blood cholesterol. Carrots enhance mental functioning and decrease the risk of cataracts and macular degeneration.

It is recommended that everyone eat 1 to 2 carrots every day.

1/2 oz	*wakame*	15 g
2 cups	shredded cabbage	500 mL
2	green onions, chopped	2
2	carrots, shredded	2
1	apple, shredded	1
1/4 cup	chopped peanuts	50 mL
1/4 cup	chopped apricots	50 mL
1/4 cup	sunflower seeds	50 mL
1/4 cup	raisins	50 mL
1/4 cup	olive oil	50 mL
2 tbsp	lemon juice	25 mL
3 tbsp	soya sauce	45 mL
2	cloves garlic, minced	2
1 tbsp	chopped candied ginger	15 mL
1/4 cup	cubed feta cheese	50 mL

1. In a medium bowl, cover *wakame* with warm water. Allow to stand for 10 minutes. Drain and set aside.

2. In a large salad bowl, toss drained *wakame* with cabbage, green onions, carrots, apple, peanuts, apricots, sunflower seeds and raisins.

3. In a small jar with a tight-fitting lid or in a bowl, combine olive oil, lemon juice, soya sauce, garlic and ginger. Shake or whisk to mix thoroughly.

4. Drizzle dressing over salad; toss to coat well. Sprinkle with feta cheese.

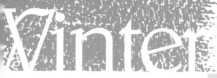
Beet and Feta Cheese Salad

Serves 4

TIP

There is no need to add salt to a dish when feta cheese is used.

VARIATIONS

Substitute: One can (19 oz [540 mL]) sliced beets for fresh beets.

Add: 2 sliced pears or apples; 1 cup (250 mL) chopped orange wedges.

4	beets, cooked and sliced	4
1/4 cup	chopped red onion	50 mL
3 tbsp	olive oil	45 mL
1 tbsp	herbed vinegar	15 mL
1 tsp	dried thyme	5 mL
1 tsp	dried marjoram	5 mL
1/2 tsp	dried rosemary	2 mL
1/4 cup	crumbled feta cheese	50 mL

1. In a salad bowl, toss beets and red onion together. Set aside.

2. In a small jar with a tight-fitting lid or a small bowl, combine oil, vinegar, thyme, marjoram and rosemary. Shake or whisk together until well mixed.

3. Pour dressing over beets and onion. Toss gently to mix. Sprinkle with feta cheese.

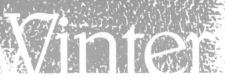

Hot Sweet Potato Salad

Serves 4 to 6

TIP

If you don't have home-made stock, use 1 cup (250 mL) of the potato cooking water in step 2.

VARIATIONS

Substitute: White potatoes for sweet potatoes.

Add: 1 cup (250 mL) cubed rutabaga in step 1.

	Preheat oven to 375° F (190° C) 9-inch (2.5 L) casserole dish, lightly oiled	
3	large sweet potatoes, cut into large chunks	3
3 tbsp	olive oil	45 mL
1	leek, white and tender green parts, sliced	1
1	onion, chopped	1
1 cup	stock	250 mL
1/4 tsp	ground cloves	1 mL
1/4 tsp	nutmeg	1 mL

1. In a large saucepan, cover potatoes with water. Bring to a boil, reduce heat and simmer for 20 minutes or until just tender. Drain.

2. In a large skillet, heat oil over medium heat. Add leek and onion; sauté until soft. Stir in stock; bring to a boil and cook, stirring occasionally, for 1 minute or until stock is thick and slightly reduced.

3. In prepared casserole dish, toss potatoes with onion mixture, cloves and nutmeg. If desired, season to taste with salt and pepper. Cover and bake in preheated oven for 30 to 40 minutes.

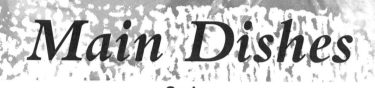

Main Dishes

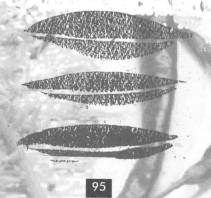

Asparagus Three-Cheese Burritos with Tomato Sauce

Makes 4 burritos

TIP

Leftover cooked vegetables work well in place of asparagas in these tasty wraps.

VARIATIONS

Substitute: Cottage cheese for ricotta cheese; Cheddar cheese or Swiss cheese for mozarella cheese; Romano cheese for Parmesan cheese; Prepared tomato sauce for sauce made in step 5.

Preheat oven to 375° F (190° C)
Baking sheet, lightly oiled

1 lb	asparagus, washed and trimmed	500 g
1 cup	ricotta cheese	250 mL
1 cup	shredded mozarella cheese	250 mL
1/4 cup	freshly grated Parmesan cheese	50 mL
3 tbsp	fresh thyme leaves	45 mL
1 tsp	sesame oil	5 mL
4	large burrito-size flour tortillas	4

Tomato Sauce

2 tbsp	olive oil	25 mL
2	cloves garlic, minced	2
1	can (19-oz [540 mL]) stewed tomatoes	1
5	sun-dried tomato halves, oil-packed, drained	5
1 cup	packed fresh chopped spinach leaves	250 mL

1. In a large pot over high heat, bring 6 cups (1.5 L) water to boil. Add asparagus and cook for 3 to 5 minutes or until tender. Drain; allow to cool.

2. Meanwhile, in a medium bowl, combine ricotta cheese, mozarella cheese, Parmesan cheese, thyme and sesame oil. Season to taste with salt and pepper if desired.

3. Spoon about 1/2 cup (125 mL) cheese mixture into center of each burrito. Divide asparagus into 4 portions; lay each portion in center of each burrito. Fold in bottom and sides of burritos and roll, allowing tips of asparagus to extend out top of roll.

4. Place burritos seam-side down on prepared baking sheet. Bake in preheated oven for 12 to 15 minutes.

Recipe continues…

FALL VEGETABLE PAELLA (PAGE 106) ➤
OVERLEAF: SEA GUMBO (PAGE 76)

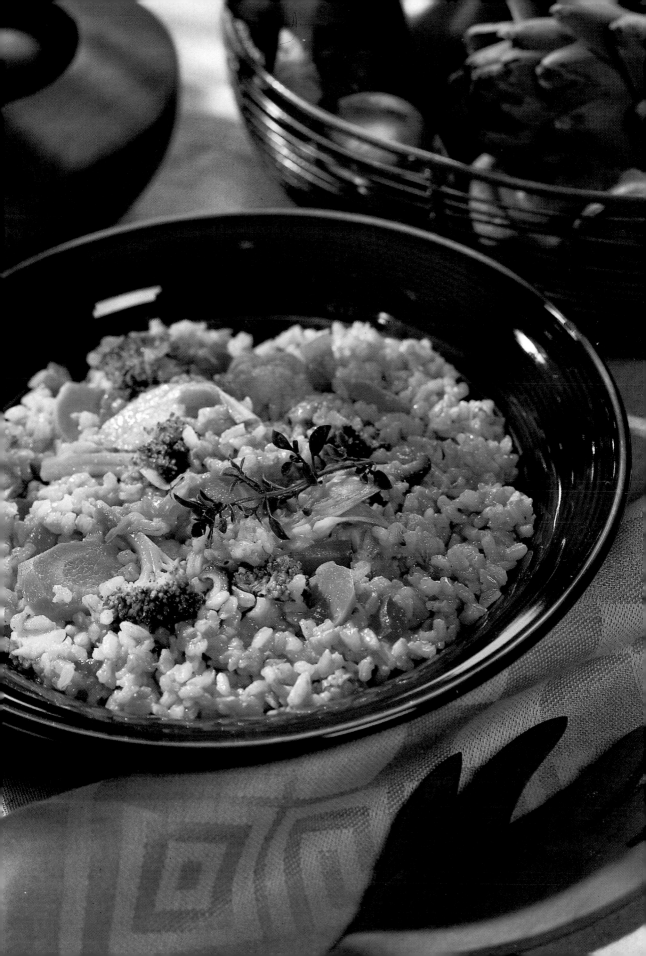

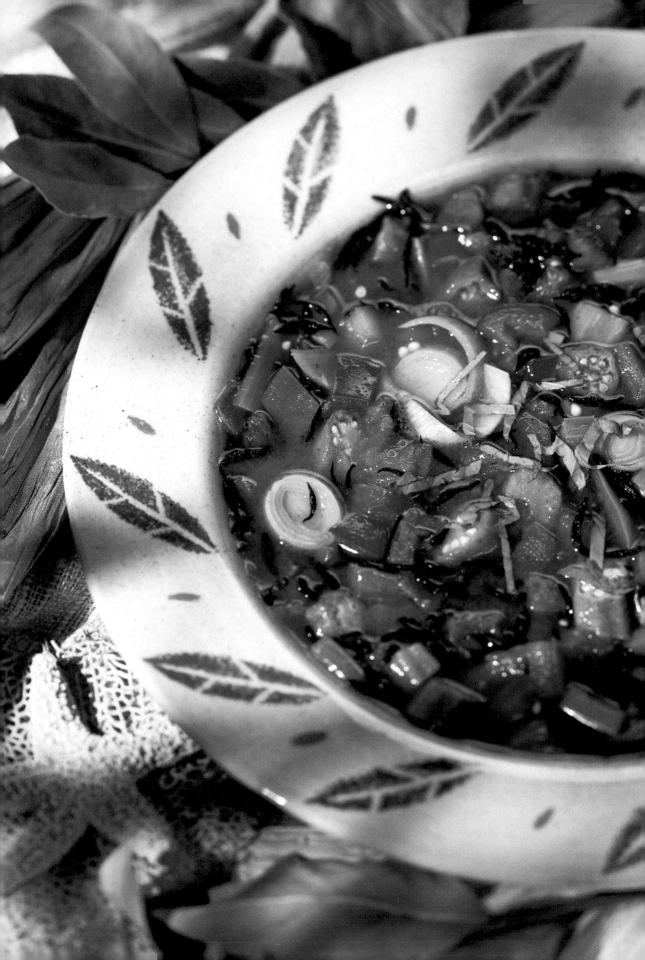

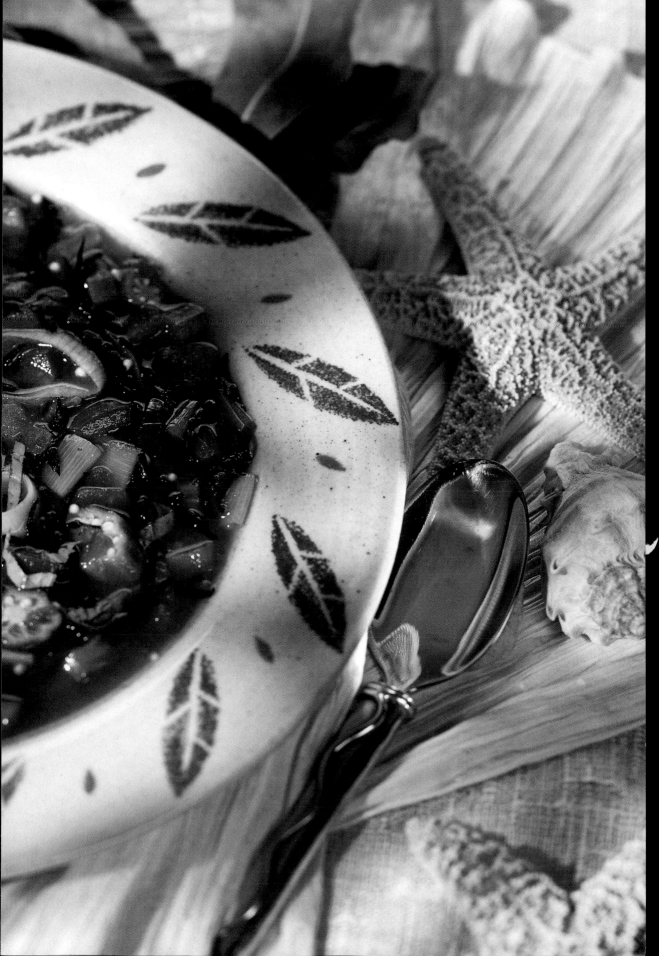

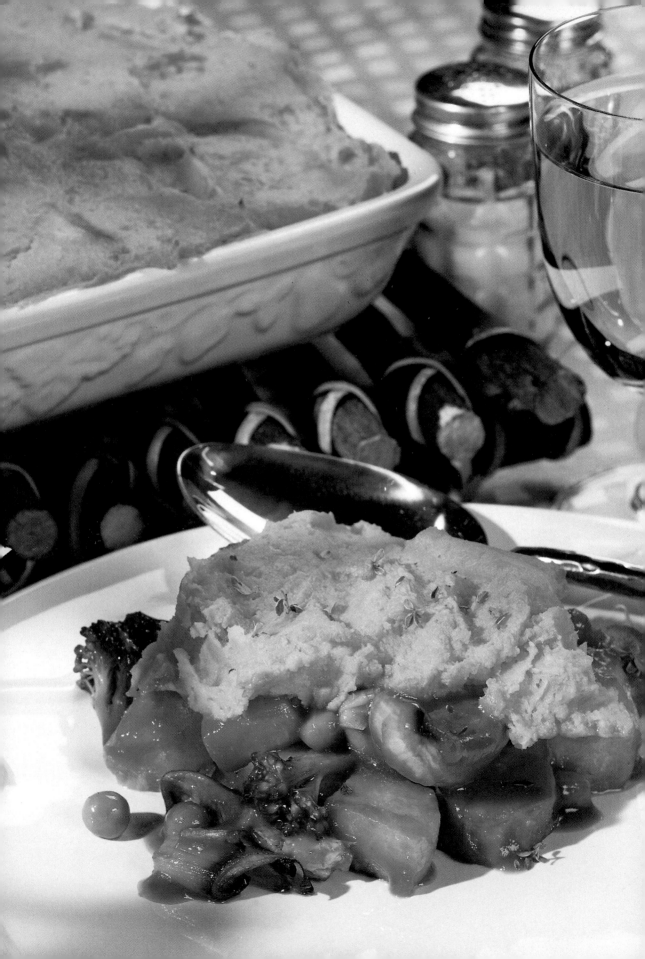

5. Meanwhile, in a medium skillet, heat oil over medium heat. Add garlic and cook for 1 minute. Stir in stewed tomatoes and sun-dried tomatoes; cover and cook for 5 minutes or until sun-dried tomatoes are soft. Stir in spinach; cook for 3 minutes or until wilted. In a food processor or blender, pureé mixture, adding up to 2 tbsp (25 mL) water, if necessary, to bring sauce to desired consistency. Return to pot and keep warm until burritos are ready.

6. Serve burritos covered in sauce or pass sauce separately.

WRAPS

Wrapping food in edible outer skins is a unique North American trend that has its roots in many diverse cultures. For us, wraps have become a new kind of sandwich — easy to make, ready to go, healthy and delicious. Look for the following wrappers in supermarkets, health/alternative stores as well as stores that supply Mexican or Middle Eastern food:

Tortilla: *A thin round flatbread, made with unleavened wheat flour or cornmeal dough, originating in Mexico. The term burrito means "large" — fajitas and tacos mean "smaller".*

Lavosh: *Delicate, flour flatbread from Armenia. Usually very large, used for rolling. 2 to 3-inch (5 to 7.5 cm) logs which are cut on the bias to make small, bite-size snacks or appetizers.*

Mountain bread: *Originating in the mountains of Middle Eastern countries, mountain bread is thick, with a bread-like texture.*

Pita: *Unleavened, eastern Mediterranean bread, with or without a "pocket".*

Chapati: *A type of Indian bread.*

Crêpe: *Thin pancake made from a thin, egg-based batter*

Healthy alternatives to refined flour wraps: *Lettuce leaves • Blanched cabbage leaves • Nori sheets*

◄ VEGETABLE POT PIE WITH SWEET POTATO TOPPING (PAGE 114)

Jambalaya

Serves 6

TIP

Use firm tofu for this recipe and put in the freezer 1 to 2 days before using.

Freezing tofu turns the color to yellow and gives it a chewy texture. Freeze tofu in the original container or drain and repackage to freeze. Squeeze thawed tofu with hands to remove extra water before using in recipes.

VARIATIONS

Substitute: Carrot and celery for dandelion and rhubarb.

Omit: Oyster sauce if unavailable.

Add: 1 to 2 tsp (5 to 10 mL) cayenne pepper, if desired.

2 tbsp	olive oil	25 mL
1	onion, chopped	1
3	cloves garlic, chopped	3
1 cup	chopped dandelion root	250 mL
1 cup	chopped rhubarb	250 mL
1/2 cup	chopped green peppers	1/2
3 tbsp	fresh thyme leaves	125 mL
2	bay leaves	2
2	dried chilies, crushed (or to taste)	2
1	can (28-oz [796 mL]) tomatoes, drained	1
2 cups	stock	500 mL
1 tsp	oyster sauce *or* fish sauce	5 mL
1 cup	long grain brown rice	250 mL
12 oz	fresh tofu, cut into 1-inch (2.5 cm) pieces *or* frozen tofu, squeezed and crumbled	500 g
2/3 cup	chopped fresh parsley	150 mL
1 tbsp	sesame oil	15 mL

1. In a large pot, heat oil over medium heat. Add onion and garlic; cook for 3 minutes or until lightly browned.

2. Stir in dandelion, rhubarb, green peppers, thyme leaves, bay leaves, chilies, tomatoes, stock and oyster sauce. Bring to a boil. Stir in rice; cover, reduce heat and simmer for 30 minutes or until rice is tender.

3. Stir in tofu, parsley and sesame oil. Season to taste with salt and pepper if desired. Discard bay leaves and serve.

Stir-Fried Vegetables with Bulgur

Serves 4

TIP

Bulgur is pre-steamed and only needs to be plumped with boiling water. If using cracked wheat, place in a saucepan and add water to cover. Simmer for 10 to 15 minutes or until tender; drain.

VARIATIONS

Substitute: Fresh cauliflower flowerets for fiddleheads; Julienned carrots for asparagus.

3/4 cup	bulgur	200 mL
1 1/2 cups	boiling water	375 mL
2 tbsp	olive oil	25 mL
1/2 cup	chopped onions	125 mL
2	cloves garlic, minced	2
2 cups	sliced fresh shiitake mushrooms	500 mL
1 cup	blanched fiddleheads	250 mL
1 cup	asparagus, cut into 1-inch (2.5 cm) pieces	250 mL
1 cup	fresh peas	250 mL
1/2 cup	chopped red bell peppers	125 mL
2 tsp	cornstarch	10 mL
3/4 cup	GINGER–CITRUS SAUCE (see recipe, page 175)	175 mL

1. In a small bowl, cover bulgur with boiling water. Set aside.

2. Meanwhile, in a wok or large skillet, heat oil over medium-high heat. Add onions and garlic; cook until lightly browned. Stir in mushrooms, fiddleheads, asparagus, peas and red pepper; cook for 3 to 5 minutes or until fiddleheads and asparagus are tender-crisp.

3. In a small bowl, whisk cornstarch into GINGER–CITRUS SAUCE. Stir sauce into vegetables; reduce heat and simmer for 3 minutes or until slightly thickened. Pour vegetables over bulgur and serve immediately.

Summer

Baked Corn-Zucchini-Beet Casseroles

Serves 6

TIP

To enjoy a taste of summer during the winter months, make extra casseroles and freeze.

VARIATIONS

Substitute: One can (10 oz [284 mL]) corn for fresh corn; Fresh turnip or 1 cup (250 mL) shredded carrots for beets; Mozarella cheese for Swiss cheese; Cooked rice or another grain for spelt.

Preheat oven to 375° F (190° C) 6 individual casserole dishes, lightly greased		
3	corn cobs	3
2 tbsp	olive oil	25 mL
1 1/2 cups	chopped zucchini	375 mL
1/2 cup	chopped red onions	125 mL
3 cups	shredded beets	750 mL
1 cup	cooked spelt kernels	250 mL
1 cup	shredded Swiss cheese	250 mL
3 tbsp	fresh thyme leaves and flowers	45 mL

1. Over a small bowl, cut kernels from cobs; set aside. Over another small bowl, run blunt end of knife down each cut cob, allowing remaining solids and corn "milk" to collect in bowl. Reserve both bowls; discard cobs.

2. In a large skillet, heat oil over medium-high heat. Add corn kernels, zucchini and onions; cook, stirring, for 5 to 6 minutes or until lightly browned and just tender. Stir in beets, spelt, cheese, thyme leaves and flowers and corn liquid.

3. Spoon into prepared casserole dishes and bake in preheated oven for 15 to 20 minutes or until cheese is melted and mixture is bubbling. Serve immediately.

CORN

The only grain indigenous to North America, corn was a major source of nourishment for the early Mesoamericans — Aztecs, Mayans, Incas and other native tribes — who cultivated it for more than 7,000 years. Indian corn became a staple of the American colonies in the 1600s, both in Virginia and Massachusetts. Within 100 years, corn had been taken back to Europe where it was used mainly as fodder for animals. Now ranked second in world grain consumption (rice is still number one), corn is one plant that has been hybridized to appeal to North America's sweet tooth.

Three sweet varieties (or genotypes) — normal sweet, sugar-enhanced and supersweet — now dominate 3% of the fresh corn market, having been developed as eating hybrids during the 1920s. All three varieties have white, yellow and bicolored kernels, but the sugar content varies. Normal, sugary and sugar-enhanced varieties have a traditional corn taste and are best eaten within one day of picking (they lose a significant amount of sugar within 24 hours). The supersweets can contain twice as much sugar (up to 44%) as old-fashioned corn and are bred so the sugars are slow to turn starchy, giving us more time to store them before they get tough.

The grain varieties of corn (yellow dent field corn accounting for over 96% of the corn grown in the U.S.) are used to make corn meal, grits and other breakfast cereals, polenta (a thick corn meal mush developed by the Italians of Tuscany, Lombardy, the Piedmont and Venetian provinces), hominy (the horny, starchy part of the corn kernel), corn oil, cornstarch, corn syrup, tortillas and breads.

Corn is a high-fiber, high-carbohydrate food that also provides some protein, B vitamins, vitamins C and E, potassium, with little sodium or fat. Corn's high phytate concentration may halt the early stages of breast cancer and cancer of the large intestine. Corn oil delivers coenzyme Q10 (co-Q10 or ubiquinone), which is essential for converting food into energy, protecting the body against free radicals, and strengthening cell membranes.

Cornsilk (Zea mays)

The stamens, or cornsilk of fresh corn is the part most important to herbalists. Cornsilk is an important ingredient — along with parsley, gravel root and hydrangea — in tinctures for kidney and bladder stones.

Actions: Demulcent; diuretic; specifically healing for urinary mucous membranes; tonic.

Summer

Barbecued Tempeh with Basil, Hyssop and Ginger

Serves 4

TIP

Commercial barbecue sauces are high in sugar, salt and preservatives. The sauce in this recipe offers the medicinal qualities of fresh, wholesome ingredients. Make double batches when tomatoes are at their peak and freeze in small amounts.

VARIATIONS

Substitute: Organic barbecue sauce (available at alternative/health stores) for barbecue sauce made in recipe; Maple syrup or molasses for ginger syrup; More or less cayenne pepper, to taste.

Preheat oven to 400° F (200° C)
Shallow baking pan, lightly greased

Barbecue Sauce

6	tomatoes	6
1	onion, quartered	1
1	head garlic	1
3 tbsp	olive oil	45 mL
1/3 cup	ginger syrup	75 mL
1/2 cup	stock	125 mL
1/4 cup	apple cider vinegar	50 mL
2 tbsp	fresh lemon juice	25 mL
1 tbsp	soya sauce	15 mL
1	can (5 1/2 oz [156 mL]) tomato paste	1
1 tsp	mustard powder	5 mL
6	fresh thyme leaves	6
1	rosemary sprig	1
1	sage sprig	1
1 tsp	cayenne pepper (or to taste)	5 mL

Tempeh

1 cup	BARBECUE SAUCE (from recipe above)	250 mL
3	basil sprigs, shredded	3
3	hyssop sprigs, shredded	3
2 tbsp	chopped candied ginger	25 mL
4	squares frozen tempeh	4
	Fresh basil or hyssop sprigs for garnish	

1. Using a sharp knife, core tomatoes, cut in half, gently squeeze out seeds and liquid. Arrange halves in prepared baking pan, cut-side down. Add onion wedges to pan.

2. Rub loose skin from outside of garlic; cut 1/4 inch (1 cm) off top and place, cut-side up, on baking pan with tomatoes and onions. Drizzle with oil.

3. Bake in preheated oven for 45 to 60 minutes until garlic is very soft and onions are browned (tomatoes will be full of liquid). Remove from oven; allow to cool slightly. Remove tomato skins.

4. Squeeze roasted garlic cloves into a food processor or blender. Add roasted onions, tomatoes with their liquid and ginger syrup; process until smooth. Season to taste with salt and pepper if desired.

5. Transfer purée to a saucepan; add stock, vinegar, lemon juice, soya sauce, tomato paste, mustard, thyme leaves, rosemary, sage and cayenne. Simmer for 15 minutes. Use sauce immediately or allow to cool. Keep in refrigerator no longer than 1 week, or freeze in 1-cup (250 mL) quantities.

6. In a small bowl, combine 1 cup (250 mL) barbecue sauce, basil, hyssop and ginger.

7. In a shallow baking dish, arrange tempeh squares in a single layer. Pour barbecue sauce over; marinate at least 2 hours at room temperature or in refrigerator overnight.

8. Preheat barbecue to medium-high. Lift squares out of marinade and grill, basting occasionally, for 3 minutes per side. Heat marinade and drizzle over tempeh to serve. Garnish with sprigs of fresh basil or hyssop.

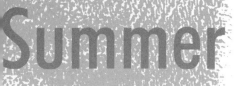

Summer

Chickpea-Herb Burgers

Makes 6 burgers

TIP

Whether grilled on the barbecue or baked in the oven, these burgers are great with all the trimmings.

VARIATIONS

Substitute: Rolled oats for spelt flakes.

	Preheat oven to 375° F (190° C) or grill to high Parchment-lined baking sheet or greased grill	
1 tbsp	vegetable oil	15 mL
1	can (19 oz [540 mL]) chickpeas, drained	1
1/2 cup	grated onions	125 mL
2	cloves garlic, minced	2
3 cups	shredded carrots	750 mL
1/2 cup	spelt flakes	125 mL
1/4 cup	unblanched almonds	50 mL
1/4 cup	sunflower seeds	50 mL
2 tbsp	flax seeds	25 mL
2 tbsp	chopped parsley	25 mL
2 tbsp	basil leaves	25 mL
1 tbsp	fresh thyme leaves	15 mL
1	egg	1

1. In a food processor or blender, purée oil, chickpeas, onion, garlic and carrots until well combined.

2. Add spelt flakes, almonds, sunflower seeds, flax seeds, parsley, basil, thyme and egg. Process until finely chopped and holding together. Season to taste with salt and pepper if desired.

3. Form mixture into 6 patties. Arrange patties on prepared baking sheet or grill. Bake in preheated oven or grill for 3 minutes per side, being careful to turn burgers gently.

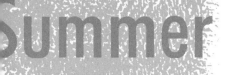

Eggplant Manicotti with Spinach Pesto Stuffing

Serves 4

Preheat oven to 375° F (190° C)
Baking sheet, lightly greased
8- by 8- inch (2 L) baking dish

2	small eggplants, cut lengthwise into 1/4-inch (1 cm) strips	2
2	cloves garlic	2
3 tbsp	toasted sunflower seeds	45 mL
1 cup	ricotta cheese	250 mL
1 cup	packed fresh basil leaves	250 mL
1/2 cup	parsley	125 mL
2 cups	packed spinach leaves	500 mL
2 tbsp	grated Parmesan cheese	25 mL
1 cup	tomato sauce	250 mL
1/2 cup	shredded mozarella cheese	125 mL

1. On prepared baking sheet, arrange eggplant strips in a single layer. (If necessary, use 2 baking sheets, broiling separately.) Broil for 3 to 5 minutes per side or until eggplant is soft and lightly browned. Allow to cool.

2. In a food processor or blender, mince garlic and sunflower seeds. Add ricotta cheese, basil, parsley, spinach and Parmesan cheese. Process until finely chopped and well blended. Season to taste with salt and pepper if desired.

3. In bottom of baking dish, spread 1/2 cup (125 mL) tomato sauce.

4. Place 2 tbsp (25 mL) filling on short end of each eggplant strip; roll up. Place rolls seam-side down in baking dish. Pour remaining tomato sauce over and top with mozarella cheese.

5. Bake in preheated oven for 25 to 30 minutes, until cheese is melted and sauce is bubbling. Serve hot.

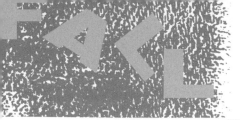

Fall Vegetable Paella

Serves 6

TIP

For a non-vegetarian dish, add 4 skinless chicken legs or breasts in step 2.

VARIATIONS

Substitute: 1 tbsp (15 mL) ground turmeric, 1 tsp (5 mL) curry powder and 2 tsp (10 mL) ground coriander for TURMERIC SPICE PASTE.

Add: One jar (6 oz [170 mL]) artichoke hearts, drained, in last 5 minutes of cooking.

3 tbsp	olive oil	45 mL
3	cloves garlic, chopped	3
1 cup	chopped onions	250 mL
1 1/2 cups	brown rice	375 mL
2 tbsp	TURMERIC SPICE PASTE (see recipe, page 132)	25 mL
2 cups	stock	500 mL
1 cup	apple juice	250 mL
2 cups	eggplant, peeled and cut into 1/2-inch (1 cm) cubes	500 mL
1/2 cup	chopped green peppers	125 mL
1/2 cup	chopped red bell peppers	125 mL
1 cup	sliced shiitake mushrooms	250 mL
1/2 cup	cauliflower florets	125 mL
1/2 cup	broccoli florets	125 mL
1/2 cup	sliced carrots	125 mL

1. In a large wok or pot, heat oil over medium heat. Add garlic and onions; cook, stirring occasionally, for 5 minutes or until soft. Stir in rice and spice paste; cook for 2 minutes.

2. Stir in stock and apple juice. Bring to a boil; cover, reduce heat and simmer for 35 minutes.

3. Stir in eggplant, green peppers, red peppers, mushrooms, cauliflower, broccoli and carrots. Cover and bring to just under a boil. Simmer gently for 10 minutes or until rice is tender and vegetables are cooked. If desired, season to taste with salt and pepper.

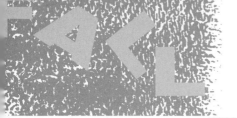

Barley and Vegetable Ragout

Serves 6

TIP

For years, pearl barley was the only type available to most North Americans. Milled six times to remove all traces of the grain's outer husk and bran layer, pearl barley is snow white and cooks in half the time — but the nutrients are missing. Look for Scotch (milled three times) or, best of all, hulled barley, the form that has the bran layer intact. Just keep in mind that hulled barley takes twice as long to cook as pearl barley.

VARIATIONS

Substitute: Turnip for parsnips; Apple juice for cider.

3 tbsp	basil pesto	45 mL
1 cup	chopped celery stalks	250 mL
2	cloves garlic, minced	2
1 cup	sliced leeks, white and tender green parts only	250 mL
3/4 cup	chopped onions	175 mL
2 cups	chopped parsnips	500 mL
1/4 cup	apple cider	50 mL
5 cups	stock	1.25 L
1 cup	hulled barley	250 mL
2 cups	sliced carrots	500 mL
1 cup	tomato sauce	250 mL
4 cups	chopped broccoli	1 L
1/4 cup	fresh chopped basil	50 mL
3 tbsp	fresh chopped parsley	45 mL
2 tbsp	fresh chopped thyme	25 mL

1. In a large bowl, toss pesto with celery, garlic, leeks, onions and parsnips.

2. In a pot, heat cider to boiling. Add pesto-coated vegetables; adjust heat and lightly boil for 3 minutes or until cider is almost gone.

3. Stir in stock; bring to a boil. Add barley; cover, reduce heat to medium-low and simmer for 40 minutes. Add carrots; cover and cook for 20 minutes or until carrots and barley are tender. If mixture seems too dry, add more stock.

4. Stir in tomato sauce, broccoli, basil, parsley and thyme. Simmer, uncovered, for 5 minutes.

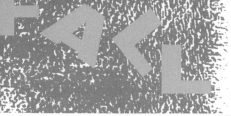

Stuffed Braised Cabbage with Potatoes

Serves 6 to 8

TIP

Locally grown fennel root is available fresh in summer and fall; but imported is available year round. Its fragrant flavor is welcome in most vegetable dishes. If fennel bulb is unavailable, substitute 1 tbsp (15 mL) dried fennel top or 1/2 cup (125 mL) chopped celery.

Preheat oven to 375° F (190° C)
Roasting pan

1	head cabbage	1
3 tbsp	butter	45 mL
1 tbsp	olive oil	15 mL
1 cup	chopped onions	250 mL
2	cloves garlic, chopped	2
1 cup	chopped carrots	250 mL
1/2 cup	chopped fennel root	125 mL
1 cup	sliced leeks, white and tender green parts only	250 mL
1 tbsp	chopped fresh sage	15 mL
2	slices whole grain bread, chopped into crumbs	2
1/2 cup	shredded Swiss cheese	125 mL
3 tbsp	grated Parmesan cheese	45 mL
1	egg	1
6	small potatoes, scrubbed	6
1 cup	plain yogurt	250 mL

1. Cut bottom stem off cabbage to sit flat. Fill a Dutch oven with water; bring to a boil. Plunge cabbage into boiling water; parboil for 6 to 8 minutes. Remove from water, drain and cut top one-third off cabbage to form a lid. Reserve cabbage cooking water.

2. Meanwhile, in a large skillet, heat butter and oil over low heat. Add onions and garlic; cook for 8 to 10 minutes or until very soft. Add carrots, fennel, leeks and sage; cook another 5 to 8 minutes or until tender.

3. Meanwhile, cut and scoop out center of parboiled cabbage, leaving about a 1-inch (2.5 cm) shell. Scoop out top lid of cabbage in the same manner. Divide scooped cabbage in half. Chop and add half to onion mixture in skillet; set remaining half aside for another use.

4. In a large bowl, combine bread crumbs, Swiss cheese, Parmesan cheese and egg with cooked vegetables. Season to taste with salt and pepper if desired. Mix well; stuff into cavity of cabbage. Top with cabbage "lid" and fasten securely with string. Place in roasting pan with 2 inches (5 cm) cabbage water; discard rest. Place potatoes around, cover pan and cook in preheated oven for 1 hour or until cabbage and potatoes are tender. Lift stuffed cabbage out of pot, remove string, slice in wedges. Serve with potatoes and a dollop of yogurt.

CABBAGE (BRASSICA OLERACEA)

Actions: *Detoxifying, diuretic, anti-inflammatory, tonic, antiseptic, restorative.*

Uses: *An excellent remedy for anemia, cabbage has also been used as a nutritive tonic to restore strength in debility and convalescence (it heals tissues by encouraging cells to proliferate). Taken as a soup, it helps protect against colds and the flu as a result of its its immune-enhancing vitamin E.*

A regular intake of cabbage prevents constipation, and has been shown to reduce the risk of cancer — particularly of the colon (because of indoles, phytochemicals found in cruciferous vegetables) — and benefits the liver. It may also reduce blood sugar, helping diabetics.

Food value:
(1 head raw cabbage)
10 g fiber
429 mg vitamin C
1143 IU vitamin A
2.72 mg niacin
0.7 mg iron
424 mg calcium
164 mg sodium
2231 mg potassium
211 mg phosphorus

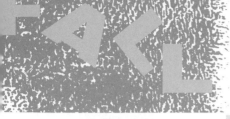

Three-Bean Enchiladas with Green Tomato and Apple Salsa

Serves 6

TIP

Make extra enchiladas and freeze for a later meal.

VARIATIONS

Substitute: Swiss cheese for Asiago cheese.

Preheat oven to 375° F (190° C)
13- by 9- inch (3 L) baking dish, lightly greased

Green Tomato and Apple Salsa

4	green tomatoes, cored and diced	4
4	apples, cored and diced	4
1 cup	chopped onions	250 mL
1/4 cup	apple juice	50 mL
1 tbsp	apple cider vinegar	15 mL
1 tbsp	brown rice syrup	15 mL
1	piece (1 inch [2.5 cm]) ginger root, minced	1
1 tbsp	mustard seeds	15 mL
1 tsp	crushed coriander seeds	5 mL
1 tsp	garam masala	5 mL
1	small dried chili pepper, crushed	1
2 tsp	ground turmeric	10 mL

Enchiladas

1	can (19-oz [540 mL]) cannellini (white kidney) beans, drained and coarsely chopped	1
1	can (19-oz [540 mL]) chickpeas, drained and coarsely chopped	1
1	clove garlic, minced	1
1/2 cup	grated Asiago cheese	125 mL
1	can (14 oz [398 mL]) refried beans	1
6	large flour tortillas	6
	Salsa	

1. In a large pot, combine tomatoes, apples, onions and apple juice. Cover and bring to a boil; reduce heat and simmer, uncovering after 5 minutes, for 25 minutes or until mixture is soft, thick and reduced to 6 cups (1.5 L).

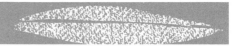

2. Stir in vinegar, brown rice syrup, ginger, mustard seeds, coriander, garam masala, chili pepper and turmeric. Simmer for another 10 minutes. Season to taste with salt and pepper if desired.

3. In a medium bowl, combine cannellini, chickpeas, garlic and cheese.

4. Spread 5 tbsp (75 mL) refried beans evenly over each tortilla to within 1 inch (2.5 cm) of edges.

5. Mound bean mixture down center of each tortilla; fold bottom and top in, then fold sides in. Place seam-side down in prepared baking dish. Cover with lid or foil. (May be made 1 day ahead and kept in refrigerator or frozen at this point; bring to room temperature before baking.)

6. Bake in preheated oven for 15 to 20 minutes or until heated through. Lift out and serve with salsa.

Winter

Black Bean Chili

Serves 4 to 6

TIP

Serve this robust chili over baked sweet or regular potatoes for a main dish or with whole grain nachos for an appetizer or party dish.

Because many of the water-soluble nutrients are in the canned liquid, try to use both the beans and the liquid from the tin. When cooking fresh beans, however, do not use cooking liquid.

VARIATIONS

Substitute: 2 cups (500 mL) any cooked beans.

2 tbsp	olive oil	25 mL
1 cup	chopped onions	250 mL
3	cloves garlic, minced	3
1 1/2 cups	chopped red bell peppers	375 mL
2	whole chilies, crushed	2
2 tsp	ground cumin	10 mL
1	can (28 oz [796 mL]) tomatoes with juice	1
1	can (19 oz [540 mL]) black beans, with liquid	1
1	can (19 oz [540 mL]) chickpeas, with liquid	1
2 tbsp	dried thyme leaves	25 mL
1 tbsp	dried savory leaves	15 mL
2 tbsp	fresh chopped parsley	25 mL

1. In a large skillet, heat oil over medium heat. Add onions, garlic, peppers and chilies; cook for 5 minutes or until soft.

2. Stir in cumin, tomatoes, black beans, chickpeas, thyme and savory. Bring to a boil; simmer for 5 minutes. Stir in parsley and serve.

BEANS AND THE DIGESTIVE SYSTEM

Dried beans are rich in oligosaccharides — complex sugars, that can't be broken down by human digestive enzymes. When you eat legumes, the oligosaccharides enter the lower intestines where they are met by bacteria which live in our systems. These bacteria eat the starches and in the process, give off gases.

The good news is that if you eat legumes on a regular basis, the system adjusts and the pain of gas is reduced. Drinking carminative herbs (cayenne, chamomile, cinnamon, clove, lavender, peppermint, parsley, rosemary, sage) in teas after meals is also helpful.

Cooking Tips to Aid Digestion

Use savory with all bean dishes as it is said to help reduce gas. Cook beans thoroughly because uncooked starch is harder to digest. Use larger amounts of water to soak, cook, drain, and rinse beans — and use fresh water often. Do not cook beans in their soaking water. Do not add salt or other seasonings during the cooking process as they toughen the bean.

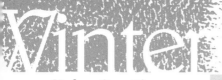

Vegetable Cakes

Makes 8 patties

TIP

For fish cakes, add 1 cup (250 mL) flaked cooked fish to the mixture in step 4. Serve as a main course with rice or whole grain and a sauce or gravy. (Check index for a variety of sauce or gravy recipes.)

VARIATIONS

Substitute: 3 parsnips for celeriac; Swiss cheese for Cheddar cheese.

	Preheat oven to 400° F (200° C) Large baking sheet, lightly oiled	
Half	rutabaga, cut into 1-inch (2.5 cm) cubes	Half
1	small celeriac, cut into 1-inch (2.5 cm) cubes	1
1/2 cup	grated old Cheddar cheese	125 mL
3 cups	fresh whole wheat bread crumbs	750 mL
2	cloves garlic, minced	2
1 cup	chopped onions	250 mL
1	1-inch (2.5 cm) piece ginger root, peeled and grated	1
1 tbsp	chopped fresh parsley	15 mL
1	egg	1
1 tbsp	honey Dijon mustard	15 mL

1. Steam rutabaga and celeriac for 25 minutes or until tender. Drain well; allow to cool.

2. Meanwhile, in a large bowl, combine cheese, 2 cups (500 mL) bread crumbs, garlic, onion, ginger and parsley.

3. In a small bowl, beat egg with mustard. Stir into cheese mixture.

4. Mash cooked rutabaga and celeriac; add to cheese mixture. Season to taste with salt and pepper. Form mixture into 8 balls.

5. Sprinkle remaining bread crumbs over a piece of waxed paper. Place balls, one at a time, on bread crumbs. Flatten to a 4-inch (10 cm) patty. Flip to coat other side.

6. On prepared baking sheet, arrange patties. Bake in preheated oven for 15 minutes per side or until lightly browned.

Winter

TIP

The complex tastes in this recipe and the fact that it can be made a day in advance make it ideal for buffet and pot luck dinners. It can also be easily put into two 10-inch (25 cm) pie pans and frozen.

If dividing this recipe between two pans, cook an extra potato for the topping.

VARIATIONS

Substitute: Dried or fresh shiitake mushrooms for black mushrooms.

Omit: Cornstarch and replace tomato juice with tomato sauce.

Vegetable Pot Pie with Sweet Potato Topping

Preheat oven to 400° F (200° C)
13- by 9- inch (3 L) baking dish

4	large dried black mushrooms	4
4 cups	chopped winter rutabaga	1 L
1 1/3 cups	chopped carrots	325 mL
1 1/3 cups	chopped parsnips	325 mL
3 tbsp	olive oil	45 mL
4 cups	chopped potatoes	1 L
3 cups	chopped onions	750 mL
6	cloves garlic, slivered	6
2 cups	chopped leeks	500 mL
2 tbsp	fresh thyme leaves	25 mL
2 tbsp	fresh chopped sage	25 mL
3	large sweet potatoes, peeled and cut into 2-inch (5 cm) pieces	3
2 tbsp	butter	25 mL
1/4 cup	plain yogurt	50 mL
1/2 tsp	nutmeg	2 mL
1 cup	broccoli florets	250 mL
1 cup	frozen peas	250 mL
2 tbsp	cornstarch	25 mL
1 cup	tomato juice	250 mL
1/2 cup	dry red wine	125 mL

1. In a medium bowl, soak mushrooms covered in 1 cup (250 mL) boiling water for 20 minutes. Drain and squeeze dry, reserving 1/2 cup (125 mL) soaking liquid. Slice mushrooms thin; set aside.

2. Meanwhile, in baking dish, combine rutabaga, carrots, parsnips and half the oil. Toss to coat well. Bake in preheated oven for 30 minutes. Add potatoes, onion, garlic, leek, thyme, sage and remaining oil. Toss to coat evenly, roast in oven for 45 to 60 minutes, stirring once, until vegetables are browned and tender. Remove from oven; reduce heat to 375° F (190° C).

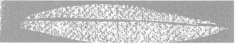

3. While vegetables are roasting, cook sweet potatoes in a large pot of boiling water for 20 minutes or until soft. Drain well and return to pot. Using a potato masher, mash potatoes, then beat in butter, yogurt, and nutmeg. Season to taste with salt and pepper. Set aside.

4. Add mushrooms, broccoli and peas to roasted vegetables in baking dish; stir to mix well.

5. In a small saucepan, mix cornstarch with 1/4 cup (50 mL) tomato juice to make a smooth paste. Whisk in remaining tomato juice, red wine and reserved mushroom soaking liquid. Bring to a simmer over medium heat; cook for 4 minutes or until sauce thickens slightly. Pour sauce over roasted vegetables; mix well. Spread mashed potato mixture evenly over top, using a spatula to smooth. (Recipe can be made ahead to this point. Freeze or store in refrigerator overnight. Return to room temperature before baking.)

6. Bake vegetable pot pie for 20 minutes or until topping is browned and vegetable mixture is tender and heated through.

Winter

Winter Vegetable Lasagna

Serves 6

TIP

For a crispy topping, omit mozzarella cheese and sprinkle with 1 cup (250 mL) store-bought muesli (or GINSENG MUESLI; see recipe page 60.)

VARIATIONS

Substitute: 4 cups (1 L) spinach for broccoli; Cooked lasagna noodles for eggplant.

Preheat oven to 400° F (200° C)
2 baking sheets, lightly oiled
9- by 13-inch (3 L) baking dish

1	large eggplant	1
3 tbsp	butter	45 mL
3	cloves garlic, finely chopped	3
1 cup	chopped onions	250 mL
5 cups	sliced shiitake mushrooms	1.25 L
1 tbsp	dried sage	15 mL
1 tbsp	dried thyme	15 mL
1 1/2 cups	stock	375 mL
1	head broccoli, chopped	1
1 cup	cottage cheese	250 mL
1/2 cup	chopped walnuts	125 mL
1/4 cup	freshly grated Parmesan cheese	50 mL
1/2 cup	shredded mozzarella cheese	125 mL
2 tbsp	chopped parsley (optional)	25 mL

1. Cut ends off eggplant, cut lengthwise into 1/4-inch (1 cm) slices. On prepared baking sheets, arrange eggplant slices in a single layer. Bake in preheated oven for 10 minutes or until slightly softened. Remove eggplant; reduce oven to 350° F (180° C).

2. Meanwhile, in a large skillet, heat butter over medium heat. Add garlic, onion, mushrooms, sage and thyme; sauté for 5 minutes, stirring occasionally. Stir in stock; bring to a boil. Cook for 5 minutes or until slightly reduced.

3. In a large bowl, mix broccoli, cottage cheese, walnuts and Parmesan cheese.

4. In prepared baking dish, spread 1 cup (250 mL) mushroom sauce. Arrange half eggplant slices in a single layer over sauce. Spread cottage cheese-broccoli mixture evenly over eggplant; spread 1 cup (250 mL) sauce over. Add remaining eggplant slices; pour remaining mushroom sauce over. Top with mozzarella cheese.

5. Cover with lid or foil; bake in preheated oven for 1 hour. Remove lid, place under broiler for 3 to 5 minutes or until golden. Sprinkle with parsley, if desired. Serve immediately.

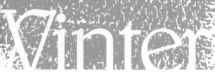
Vinter

Makes 10 wraps

TIP

This makes enough filling for 10 large wraps so if you don't have a large crowd to feed, make half the recipe or freeze leftover filling.

VARIATIONS

Substitute: Sour cream for yogurt; 1 1/2 cups (375 mL) cooked lentils or chickpeas for lima beans.

Omit: Olives and lettuce, if desired.

Cracked Wheat and Lima Bean Wrap

2 tbsp	olive oil	25 mL
1 cup	chopped onions	250 mL
2	cloves garlic, minced	2
1 cup	chopped celery	250 mL
2 tbsp	finely chopped preserved ginger	25 mL
1 tsp	ground cumin	5 mL
1 tbsp	ground turmeric	15 mL
1 cup	cracked wheat	250 mL
3 tbsp	fresh lemon juice	45 mL
1	can (28 oz [796 mL]) stewed tomatoes	1
1	can (19 oz [540 mL]) lima beans, drained and coarsely chopped	1
2/3 cup	plain yogurt	150 mL
10	large flour tortillas	10
1 cup	sliced black olives	250 mL
2 cups	shredded lettuce	500 mL

1. In a large skillet, heat oil over medium-low heat. Cook onions and garlic for 10 minutes or until soft. Add celery; cook, stirring often, for 3 minutes. Add ginger, cumin and turmeric; cook for 2 minutes.

2. Stir in cracked wheat, lemon juice and tomatoes, breaking up tomatoes with back of a spoon. Cover; simmer over low heat for 20 minutes or until liquid is absorbed and wheat is tender.

3. Remove from heat; stir in lima beans. Season to taste with salt and pepper. Allow to cool to room temperature or store in refrigerator for up to 3 days.

4. Spread 1 tbsp (15 mL) yogurt on each tortilla. Spoon about 1/2 cup (125 mL) filling down center of each wrap. Top with 1 rounded tbsp (15 mL) olives and 3 tbsp (45 mL) lettuce. Fold bottom up and both sides in, leaving top open. Fold in half. Serve slightly warm.

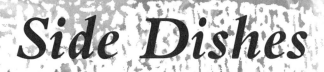

Side Dishes

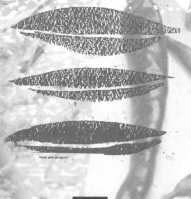

Braised Spring Vegetables with Citrus Dressing

Serves 4

TIP

Use carrots, squash, regular peas, turnips or any of your favorite vegetables in this light, spring vegetable dish.

VARIATIONS

Substitute: Water for stock; 3 domestic leeks, cleaned and sliced in half lengthwise and cut into 2-inch (5 cm) pieces for wild leeks; Regular thyme for lemon thyme.

Omit: Lemongrass if not available.

4 cups	stock	1 L
8	small new potatoes, scrubbed	8
1	onion, quartered	1
20	whole wild leeks, trimmed	20
1 lb	asparagus, cut into 2-inch (5 cm) pieces	500 g
1 cup	snow peas	250 mL
1 tbsp	olive oil	15 mL
2	cloves garlic, finely chopped	2
2 tbsp	fresh chopped lemon thyme	25 mL
1	stalk fresh lemongrass, lightly pounded and cut in half	1
1 tbsp	maple syrup	15 mL
2 tbsp	lemon juice	25 mL
1 tbsp	grated lemon zest	15 mL

1. In a large skillet with lid, bring stock to a boil. Add potatoes; reduce heat to simmer and cook potatoes, covered, for 5 minutes. Add onion and leeks, cook for 3 minutes. Add asparagus; cook for 2 minutes. Add snow peas; cook for 2 minutes. The vegetables should be tender-crisp.

2. Drain vegetables, reserving 1 cup (250 mL) stock for dressing. (Set aside remainder for another use.) Transfer vegetables to a serving platter; keep warm while making dressing. Wipe skillet dry.

3. In same skillet, heat oil over medium-low heat. Add garlic and cook for 2 minutes or until soft. Stir in thyme, lemongrass and reserved stock; bring to a boil, adjust heat to keep lightly boiling for 5 minutes or until liquid is reduced by half. Stir in maple syrup, lemon juice and lemon zest. Simmer for another 2 minutes. Season to taste with salt and pepper if desired. Remove lemongrass and drizzle sauce over braised vegetables or serve on the side.

LEMON HERBS

The easiest way to add the tangy temperament and invigorating perfume of lemon is by chopping lemon herbs into dishes. Used with cooked rice, pasta, chicken, fish, stir-fries, jellies, jams, beverages, cakes, breads, muffins, dressings and sauces, lemon herbs add a fresh, clean note.

Golden lemon thyme
(Thymus x "Aureus") *A hardy, small bush with yellow colored leaves. The flavor is a blend of lemon and earthy thyme.*

Lemon balm
(Melissa officinalis) *a hardy perennial, easy to grow (except in the humid South), opposite, oval, strongly lemon-scented leaves grow on thin, square, 2-foot (60 cm) long stems.*

Lemon basil
(Ocimum basilicum 'Citriodorum') *A fragrant annual, grown as regular basil, smooth, pale green, oval, lemony leaves are smaller than those of sweet basil.*

Lemongrass
(Cymbopogon citratus) *A tropical grass native to Southeast Asia with tufts of green, spear-shaped leaves that grow to 3 feet (90 cm). The white bulbous end is crushed or smashed before adding to soups, stews or other dishes and removed at the end of cooking.*

Lemon-scented geranium
(Pelargonium "Lemon Crispum") *An edible scented geranium with leaves that have a true lemon scent, it can be used whole, to line cake tins or shredded and added to baked goods and sauces.*

Lemon verbena
(Aloysia triphylla) *A fast-growing shrub native to South America; grows over 6 feet (180 cm) tall in tropical areas (hardy to zone 9); long, pointed leaves grow on woody erect stems. The intense, sweet lemon scent persists strongly in baked goods.*

Scalloped Turnips with Potatoes and Onion

Serves 4 to 6

Preheat oven to 350° F (180° C) 9-inch (2.5 L) casserole dish, buttered		
3 cups	thinly sliced potatoes	750 mL
1 1/3 cups	thinly sliced sweet potatoes	325 mL
1/4 cup	basil pesto	50 mL
3 cups	thinly sliced fresh turnips	750 mL
1 cup	thinly sliced onions	250 mL
1/4 cup	whole wheat flour	50 mL
1 cup	stock	250 mL
1/2 cup	shredded mozzarella cheese	125 mL

1. In a large bowl, toss potatoes and sweet potatoes with pesto, coating well. If desired, season to taste with salt.

2. Spread one-third of potatoes in prepared casserole dish. Cover with half the turnip slices and half the onion slices. Sprinkle with 2 tbsp (25 mL) flour. Pour 1/2 cup (125 mL) stock over.

3. Repeat procedure in step 2, ending with a layer of potatoes. Top with cheese; cover with lid or aluminum foil. Bake in preheated oven for 30 minutes. Remove lid and bake for another 20 to 30 minutes or until vegetables are tender and top is brown.

TURNIP

A member of the cruciferous family, the leaves and root of the turnip plant are edible. Turnip has a beneficial effect on the urinary system, purifies the blood and aids in the elimination of toxins. Both the root and green tops are high in glucosinolates which are thought to block the development of cancer.

Actions: tonic, decongestant, bactericidal, diuretic.

How to use in cooking: grated raw into salads — in particular, cabbage salads. Chop one turnip and add to recipes where onion is used. Boil and mash with carrots (saving the cooking water as stock) and use as a vegetable accompaniment.

Asparagus with Spring Sauce

Serves 4

TIP

Use this light, tangy cream sauce with any spring or summer vegetable or tossed with pasta for a low-fat main dish.

The sauce can be prepared up to 3 days in advance and kept refrigerated.

VARIATIONS

Substitute: Domestic leeks for wild leeks; French sorrel for sheep sorrel; Swiss chard or spinach for dandelion.

2 tbsp	butter	25 mL
1 cup	chopped wild leeks, stalks and leaves	250 mL
2 cups	chopped sheep sorrel	500 mL
2 cups	chopped dandelion leaves	500 mL
1 cup	stock	250 mL
1 tbsp	maple syrup	15 mL
1 cup	yogurt	250 mL
1/2 tsp	nutmeg	2 mL
1 1/2 lbs	fresh asparagus	750 g

1. In a medium saucepan, heat butter over medium heat. Add leeks and sauté for 10 minutes or until soft. Stir in sheep sorrel and dandelion leaves; cook until wilted. Pour in stock and maple syrup; bring to a boil. Reduce heat and simmer, uncovered, for 10 minutes or until liquid is reduced by half. Allow to cool. Stir in yogurt and nutmeg. Season to taste with salt and pepper if desired.

2. Meanwhile, steam or parboil asparagus for 2 to 4 minutes or until tender-crisp. Serve with sauce immediately or at room temperature.

SHEEP SORREL (RUMEX ACETOSELIA)

French sorrel (rumex scutatus), is a regular feature on spring menus because of its slightly acid-tasting leaves and the fact that it is always the first green to appear in domestic gardens. A close relative, sheep sorrel is found in waste urban areas and along country roads and is easily available all season long; it makes a delicious green for salads or soups.

Use: traditionally used for fevers, inflammation, diarrhea, excessive menstruation and cancer, sheep sorrel is one of the four ingredients of the Essiac® anti-cancer remedy. It can be used fresh as you would spinach or dried and blended with other herbs for teas.

Stuffed Squash Flowers

Serves 4

TIP

Any large edible flower — squash, zucchini, pumpkin, day lily — is suitable for stuffing and baking in this appetizer or side dish.

VARIATIONS

Substitute: Prepared honey mustard for pesto; Mozzarella cheese or Cheddar cheese for Parmesan cheese.

Preheat oven to 350° F (180° C)
Baking dish, lightly oiled

2 cups	cooked rice	500 mL
1/4 cup	pesto (basil, calendula or any other)	50 mL
1/4 cup	freshly grated Parmesan cheese	50 mL
1/4 cup	finely chopped red or green bell pepper	50 mL
1	egg, slightly beaten	1
8	squash flowers, cleaned with stamen removed	8

1. In a medium bowl, combine rice, pesto, Parmesan cheese, pepper and egg. Season to taste with salt and pepper, if desired Spoon into squash flowers.

2. Place stuffed flowers into prepared baking dish; cover and bake in preheated oven for 20 minutes or until stuffing is set.

Golden Cauliflower with Split Peas

3/4 cup	dried split green peas	175 mL
2 tbsp	olive oil	25 mL
1 tsp	cumin seed	5 mL
1 tbsp	minced ginger root	15 mL
1 tbsp	minced turmeric root	15 mL
1	1-inch (2.5 cm) piece cinnamon root, crushed	1
1	1-inch (2.5 cm) piece dried licorice root, crushed	1
1	small cauliflower, cut into florets	1
1 cup	chopped scapes	250 mL

1. In a medium saucepan, cover split peas with 2 cups (500 mL) water. Cover and bring to a boil; reduce heat and simmer for 15 to 20 minutes or until peas are just tender. Drain.

2. Meanwhile, in a large skillet or wok, heat oil over medium heat. Add cumin, ginger, turmeric, cinnamon and licorice; toast for 1 minute or until seeds turn brown.

3. Add cauliflower and cook, covered, over medium-low heat for 10 minutes, stirring occasionally. Add scapes; replace cover and cook for 5 to 10 minutes or until vegetables are just tender. Stir in cooked peas and warm through.

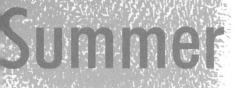

Tomatoes Stuffed with Basil and Shiitake Mushrooms

Serves 4

TIP

Herbalists use basil (*ocimum basilicum*) for these actions: antidepressant, antiseptic, prevents vomiting, stimulates the adrenal cortex, carminative, febrifuge, expectorant, soothes itching.

VARIATIONS

Substitute: Spelt or kamut for rice; 1/4 cup (50 mL) pesto sauce for fresh basil; Bread crumbs or muesli (or GINSING MUESLI; see recipe page 60) for Parmesan cheese.

Preheat oven to 350° F (180° C)
Small baking dish, lightly greased

4	large tomatoes, firm and ripe	4
1 tbsp	butter	15 mL
1 tbsp	olive oil	15 mL
3	cloves garlic, minced	3
1 cup	chopped onions	250 mL
1/2 cup	thinly sliced fresh shiitake mushrooms	125 mL
1 cup	cooked rice	250 mL
1/2 cup	chopped fresh basil	125 mL
1 tbsp	chopped fresh thyme leaves	15 mL
1 tbsp	chopped fresh hyssop	15 mL
1/4 cup	freshly grated Parmesan cheese	50 mL

1. Core tomatoes and slice 1/2 inch (1 cm) off top. Set tops aside. Scoop out seeds and juice to form a cavity. Chop tomato tops and inside flesh; set aside. Place tomatoes in prepared baking dish; set aside.

2. In a medium saucepan, heat butter and oil over medium heat. Add garlic, onions and mushrooms; sauté for 5 minutes or until softened. Add reserved chopped tomato, rice, basil, thyme and hyssop; cook, stirring well, for 1 minute. If desired, season to taste with salt and pepper.

3. Divide stuffing evenly into 4 portions; stuff into tomato cavities. Sprinkle each tomato with cheese.

4. Bake in preheated oven for 10–15 minutes or until cheese melts and tomatoes begin to soften.

TOMATOES

Phytochemistry: Lypocene, found in red, orange and yellow fruits and vegetables, is the parent substance from which all natural carotenoid pigments are derived. Italian researchers have discovered that people who consume more raw tomatoes on average can decrease the risk of developing gastrointestinal cancers. Ongoing research indicates that lycopene (relatively rare in foods but high in tomatoes) and glutathione, two powerful antioxidants, can reduce the risk of macular degenerative disease, serum lipid oxidation and cancers of the lung, bladder, skin and cervix. Lycopene is also thought to help maintain mental and physical functioning. It is absorbed by the body

Continued on facing page...

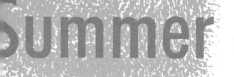

Roasted Peppers with Wild Rice and Walnuts

Serves 6

TIP

Use this stuffing with baked, whole potatoes, zucchini or eggplant for an easy, make-ahead appetizer or side dish.

VARIATIONS

Substitute: Green bell peppers for red bell peppers; 1/4 cup (50 mL) shredded basil for basil pesto; Any pesto for basil pesto.

	Preheat oven to 400° F (200° C) Baking pan, lightly greased	
6	red bell peppers, cored and cut into half	6
3 tbsp	olive oil	45 mL
4	cloves garlic, minced	4
3 cups	chopped shiitake mushrooms	750 mL
2 cups	chopped seeded tomatoes	500 mL
1/2 cup	basil pesto	125 mL
2	anchovies, finely chopped	2
1 cup	cooked wild rice	250 mL
1/4 cup	chopped walnuts	50 mL
2 tbsp	Parmesan cheese	25 mL

1. On prepared baking pan, arrange peppers cut-side down. Bake on top rack of preheated oven for 10 minutes or until slightly softened. Remove from oven, flip peppers over so cut sides are up.

2. Meanwhile, in a medium-sized skillet, heat oil over medium heat. Add garlic and mushrooms; cook until soft. Stir in tomato, pesto, anchovies and rice. If desired, season to taste with salt and pepper.

3. Divide rice mixture into pepper halves. Return to oven and bake for 10 minutes.

4. Remove from oven; sprinkle with walnuts and Parmesan cheese. Bake for 5 to 10 minutes or until peppers are very soft. Serve warm.

more efficiently when tomatoes are processed into juice, sauce and paste.

According to scientists at the Rambam Medical Centre in Haifa, Israel, when these tomato products are combined with cold-pressed extra virgin olive oil, they become even more beneficial.

Tomatoes also contain glutamic acid, a naturally occurring amino acid that is converted in the human system to gamma-amino butyric acid (GABA). GABA is a calming agent, known to be effective for kidney hypertension. Hence, tomato soup could be the answer to calming your nerves.

Celery Root and Potatoes au Gratin

Serves 6

TIP

Celery root, also called celeriac, is a variety of celery grown for its roots instead of the stalks. The flavor is a subtle anise. It can be substituted for potatoes in most recipes. Do not peel or cut the celery root until just before cooking as it darkens when exposed to air. As with apples, submerging in water with 2 to 3 tbsp (25 to 45 mL) lemon juice keeps cut pieces from turning brown.

VARIATIONS

Substitute: Turnips or kohlrabi for celery root; 1 cup (250 mL) muesli (or GINSING MUESLI; see recipe, page 60) for whole wheat topping.

Preheat oven to 350° F (180° C)
Large casserole dish, greased

5	small potatoes, each cut into 4 wedges	5
1	celery root, cut into 1/2-inch (1 cm) cubes	1
2 tbsp	butter	25 mL
2 tbsp	olive oil	25 mL
1 1/2 cups	sliced leeks	375 mL
1 cup	chopped onions	250 mL
5 tbsp	spelt flour	75 mL
1/2 tsp	cayenne pepper	2 mL
1/2 tsp	dry mustard	2 mL
1/2 cup	shredded Swiss cheese	125 mL

Topping (optional)

3	slices wholewheat bread, crusts removed, torn into pieces	3
1 tbsp	butter	15 mL
1/2 cup	freshly grated Parmesan cheese	125 mL

1. In a large saucepan, cover potatoes and celery root with water; bring to a boil. Reduce heat and simmer for 5 to 10 minutes or until just tender. Drain cooked vegetables, reserving 2 cups (500 mL) of cooking liquid.

2. In a large saucepan, heat butter and oil. Add leeks and onions; cook for 10 minutes or until soft. Stir in flour, cayenne pepper and mustard. Cook, stirring, for 2 minutes. Stir in reserved cooking liquid; simmer gently for 2 to 3 minutes or until thickened.

3. Remove from heat; stir in Swiss cheese with potato-and-celery root mixture. If desired, season to taste with salt and pepper. Mix well. Transfer to prepared casserole. The dish is now ready to serve; topping and baking are optional.

4. Topping: In a food processor or blender, process bread, butter and cheese until fine and crumbly. Spread on top of casserole. Bake for 20 to 25 minutes or until top is crisp and mixture is bubbling.

GOLDEN CAULIFLOWER WITH SPLIT PEAS (PAGE 125) ➤

OVERLEAF: FETTUCCINE AND FIDDLEHEADS IN THYME VINAIGRETTE (PAGE 140)

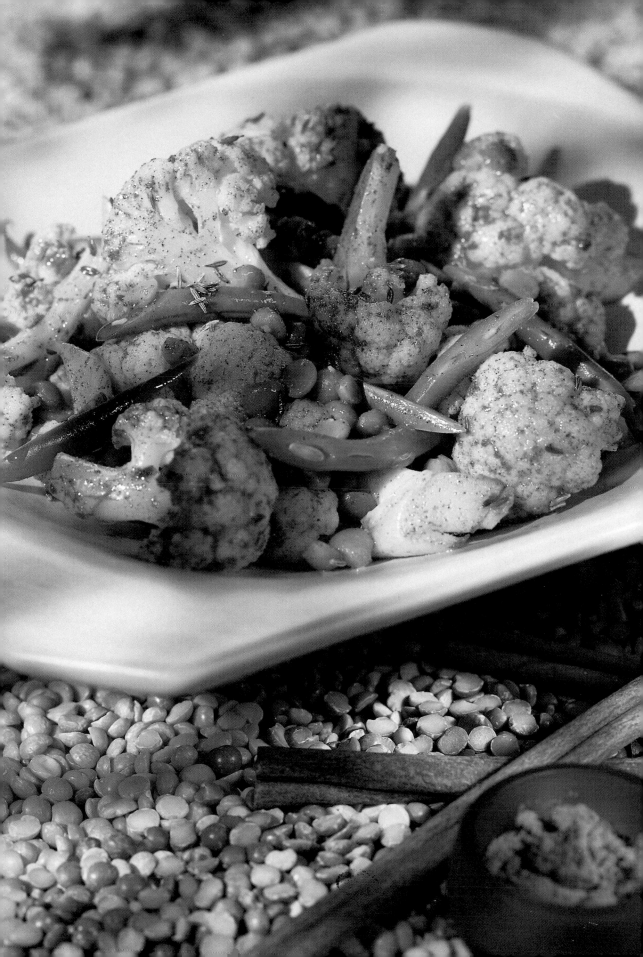

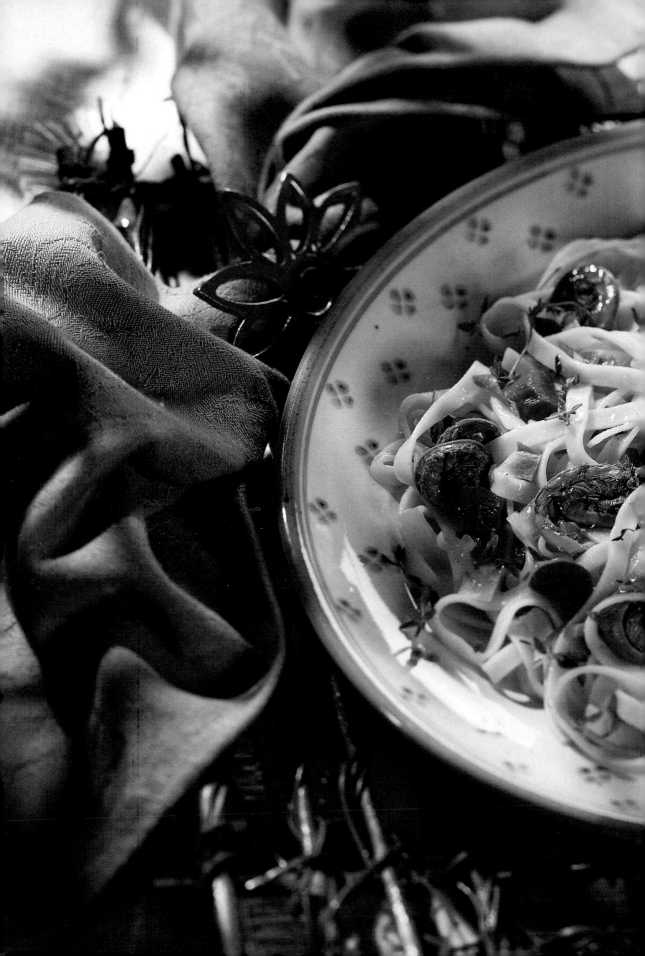

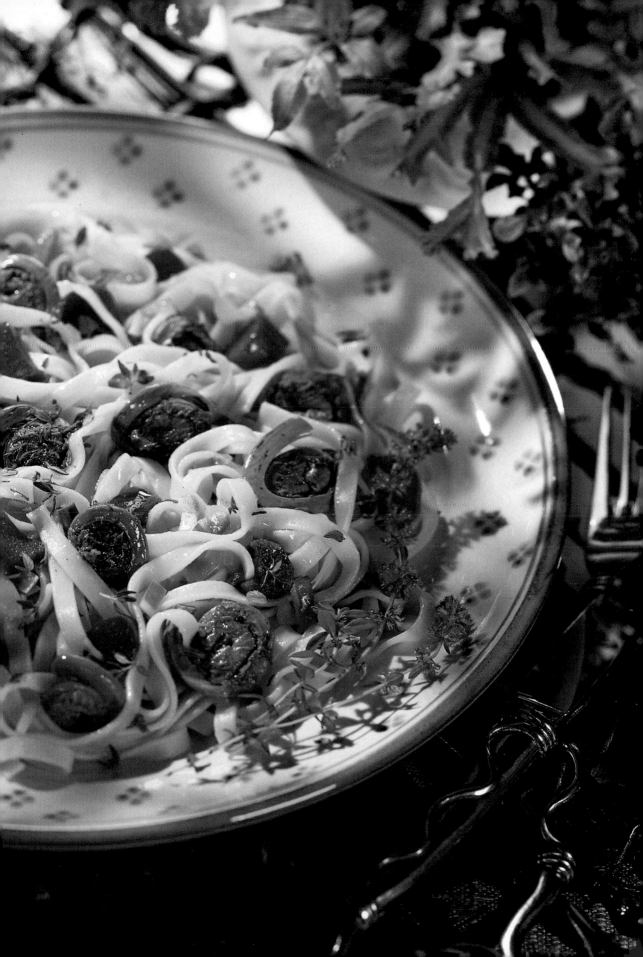

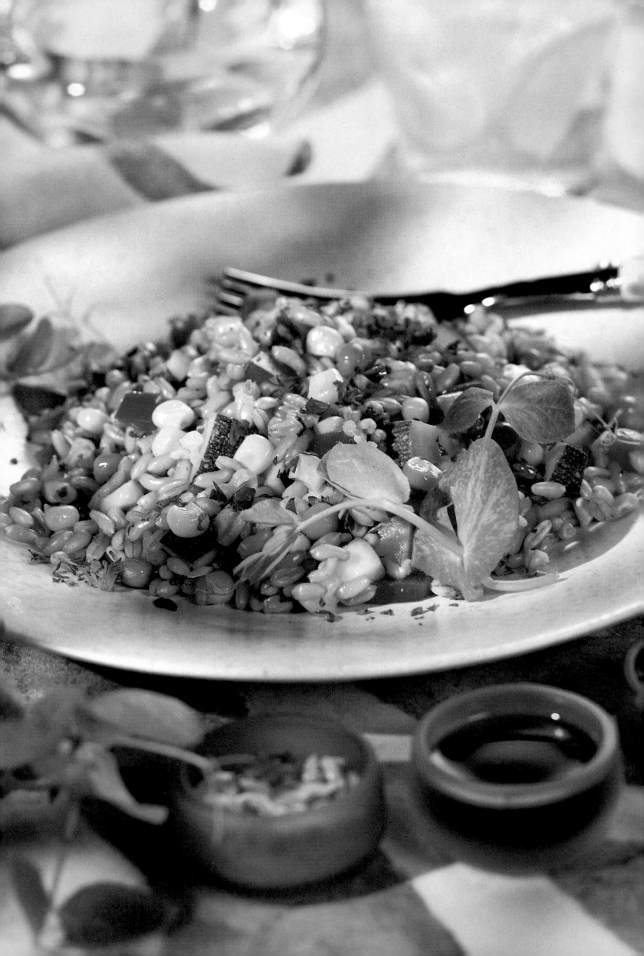

Baked Moroccan Squash

Serves 4 to 6

TIP

Any of the fall squashes — turban, acorn, pattypan, butternut — are suitable for this recipe.

VARIATIONS

Substitute: 1 tsp (5 mL) dried ground cardamom for seeds, 1 tsp (5 mL) dried crumbled sage leaves for fresh sage.

Preheat oven to 350° F (180° C)
Dutch oven or ovenproof skillet with lid

3 tbsp	olive oil	45 mL
4	cloves garlic, minced	4
1	large onion, chopped	1
2 tsp	ground cumin	10 mL
1 tsp	cardamom seeds, crushed	5 mL
1 tbsp	curry powder	15 mL
1 tbsp	garam masala	15 mL
1 tbsp	chopped fresh sage	15 mL
1 tbsp	minced crystalized ginger	15 mL
3/4 cup	stock	175 mL
1/2 cup	applesauce	125 mL
2 lbs	squash, cut into 1-inch (2.5 cm) cubes	1 kg
1/2 cup	raisins	125 mL
1/2 cup	sliced dried apricots	125 mL
1/2 cup	pitted whole prunes	125 mL

1. In a Dutch oven, heat oil over medium heat. Add garlic and onion; cook for 7 minutes or until soft. Add cumin, cardamom, curry powder, garam masala, sage and ginger. Cook, stirring, for 1 minute. Stir in stock, scraping up brown bits from bottom of pan.

2. Add applesauce, squash, raisins, apricots and prunes. Stir well to coat squash cubes. Season to taste with salt and pepper if desired. Bake, covered, in preheated oven for 45 minutes or until squash is tender.

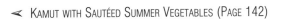

◄ KAMUT WITH SAUTÉED SUMMER VEGETABLES (PAGE 142)

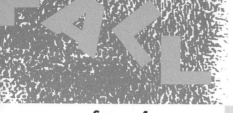

Baked Potatoes with Caramelized Onions and Leek

TIP

Use sweet potatoes or a mixture of white and sweet potatoes with turnip.

VARIATIONS

Substitute: Cheddar cheese or Swiss cheese for Romano cheese.

	Preheat oven to 400° F (200° C) Large baking pan, lightly greased	
2	large Vidalia or Spanish onions, cut into 8 wedges	2
1	large leek, white and tender green parts, cut into 2-inch (5 cm) pieces	1
8	cloves garlic, peeled	8
2 tbsp	balsamic vinegar	25 mL
3 tbsp	olive oil	45 mL
1 tbsp	fresh thyme leaves	15 mL
4	medium potatoes, scrubbed and pricked	4
1/4 cup	grated Romano cheese	50 mL

1. In a large bowl, combine onions, leek, garlic, vinegar, oil and thyme. If desired, season to taste with salt and pepper. Spread on prepared baking pan.

2. Add whole potatoes to pan. Roast in preheated oven for 20 minutes, stirring onions occasionally. Reduce heat to 375° F (190° C), roast for another 25 to 35 minutes or until onions are golden and potatoes are soft.

3. Remove from oven; split potatoes in half. Divide onions onto baked potato halves; sprinkle each with 1 tbsp (15 mL) Romano cheese. Serve warm.

LEEKS

Welsh legend holds that in the 7th century, the Welsh leader Cadwallon battled Edwin, King of Northumbria. Cadwallon won, due in great part to the odor of leeks from his soldiers' helmets — it helped him distinguish them from the enemy. To this day, the Welsh wear a leek in their hats on March 1st, the honorary day of St. David. A centu-ry earlier, it is said, leeks saved King Arthur and his army from starvation when they were besieged by the Saxons.

Actions: expectorant, diuretic, relaxant, laxative, antiseptic, digestive, hypotensive.

Uses: Easily digested, leeks are taken in a broth as a tonic, expecially during con-valescence from illness. Their warming, expectorant and stimulating properties pro-vide relief for sore throats, colds and chest infections. Used in food with onions and garlic, leeks add to the anti-cancer and heart-help-ing properties of those alli-ums. Add one chopped leek to any dish that calls for onion.

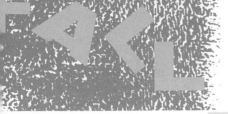

Tomatoes and Goat Cheese with Pesto and Balsamic Vinegar

Serves 6

TIP

Any pesto will work in this dish. Try ROASTED GARLIC AND RED PEPPER (see recipe, page 59) or CORIANDER PESTO or CALENDULA PESTO (see recipes, pages 170 to 172).

VARIATIONS

Substitute: Feta cheese for soft goat cheese.

1/2 cup	pesto (see Tip, at left)	125 mL
6	tomatoes, cored and sliced	6
4.5 oz	soft goat cheese	140 g
1/4 cup	balsamic vinegar	50 mL

1. Spread 1/2 tsp (2 mL) pesto on each slice of tomato. Arrange on a serving platter. If desired, season to taste with salt and pepper. Crumble cheese over and drizzle with vinegar.

2. Allow to stand for 30 minutes or longer. Serve at room temperature.

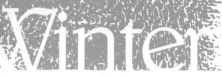

Braised Winter Vegetables

Serves 4 to 6

TIP

Add 1 can (19 oz [540 mL]) chickpeas or lima beans, drained, and serve over whole grains for a high-protein dish.

VARIATIONS

Substitute: 2 tbsp (25 mL) commercial curry blend spice for spice paste; Broccoli spears for Brussels sprouts; 1 tbsp (15 mL) dried powdered turmeric for fresh turmeric root.

Add: 1 can (19 oz [540 mL]) chickpeas, lima beans or kidney beans, drained, 5 minutes before the end of cooking time; 1 cup (250 mL) tempeh cubes in step 3.

Spice Paste

1 tbsp	olive oil	15 mL
1	1-inch (2.5 cm) cinnamon stick	2.5 cm
2	cloves garlic, finely chopped	2
1 tsp	whole coriander seeds	5 mL
1/2 tsp	ground cumin	2 mL
1	2-inch (5 cm) piece turmeric root, peeled and finely chopped	1
1	1-inch (2.5 cm) piece ginger root, peeled and finely chopped	1
1	whole clove	1

Vegetables

2 tbsp	olive oil	25 mL
1	onion, chopped	1
1	can (28 oz [796 mL] tomatoes	1
1 cup	stock	250 mL
1	sweet potato, peeled and cut into 1/2-inch (1 cm) cubes	1
1 cup	chopped carrots	250 mL
1 cup	chopped parsnips	250 mL
Half	rutabaga, peeled and cut into 1/2-inch (1 cm) cubes	Half
2 cups	Brussel sprouts, halved	500 mL

1. In a small skillet, heat 1 tbsp (15 mL) olive oil over medium heat. Add cinnamon, garlic and coriander seeds; gently toast, stirring, for 2 minutes. Transfer to a clean coffee grinder. Add cumin, turmeric, ginger and clove; grind into a rough paste.

2. In a large pot, heat 2 tbsp (25 mL) olive oil over low heat. Add chopped onion and spice paste; sweat for 8 minutes or until soft and fragrant. Increase heat to medium; add tomatoes and their juice, simmer for 2 minutes. Stir in stock and bring to a boil.

3. Add sweet potato, carrots, parsnips, rutabaga and Brussel sprouts. If desired, season to taste with salt and pepper. Reduce heat to simmer; cover and cook for 25 to 35 minutes or until vegetables are tender-crisp.

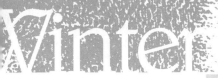

Fruit-Stuffed Roasted Eggplant

Serves 4

TIP

Though commonly thought of as a vegetable, eggplant is actually a fruit.

VARIATIONS

Substitute: 2 small acorn squash for eggplants (increase the baking time to 1 hour); 2 large zucchini for eggplants

Preheat oven to 350° F (180° C)
10-inch (3 L) casserole with lid, lightly greased

2	small eggplants, about 1 lb (500 g) each	2
1 1/2 cups	chopped apples	375 mL
1/2 cup	coarsely chopped prunes	125 mL
1/4 cup	coarsely chopped dried apricots	50 mL
2 tbsp	raspberry vinegar	25 mL
1	onion, chopped	1
2 tsp	dried lavender buds	10 mL
1/2 cup	applesauce	125 mL
2 tbsp	butter	25 mL

1. Cut eggplants in half lengthwise. Scoop out seeds, making eggplants hollow. In prepared casserole dish, arrange eggplant halves, cut-side up. Set aside.

2. In a medium bowl, combine apples, prunes, apricots, vinegar, onion, lavender and applesauce. If desired, season to taste with salt. Divide fruit mixture into 4 portions; spoon into eggplant halves. Spread one-quarter of the butter over fruit for each portion.

3. Cover and bake in preheated oven for 50 to 60 minutes or until tender.

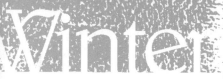
Calendula-Glazed Parsnips

Serves 4

TIP

If you have homemade herbed honey, use it in this recipe.

Parsnips are believed to have anti-cancer properties. Use them in soups, stews and chopped in stir-fries and other dishes with carrots and potatoes.

VARIATIONS

Substitute: 1 tbsp (15 mL) saffron or any dried herb for calendula petals; White vinegar for herbed vinegar.

1 lb	parsnips, cut into sticks	500 g
2 tbsp	butter	15 mL
3 tbsp	honey	45 mL
2 tbsp	dried calendula petals	25 mL
2 tbsp	herbed vinegar	25 mL

1. Steam parsnips for 6 minutes or until tender-crisp.

2. In a large skillet, heat butter over medium heat. Add parsnips; cook, stirring, for 3 minutes or until lightly brown.

3. Stir in honey, calendula and vinegar. Cook for another 1 to 2 minutes or until glaze is thick and parsnips are well coated. If desired, season to taste with salt and pepper.

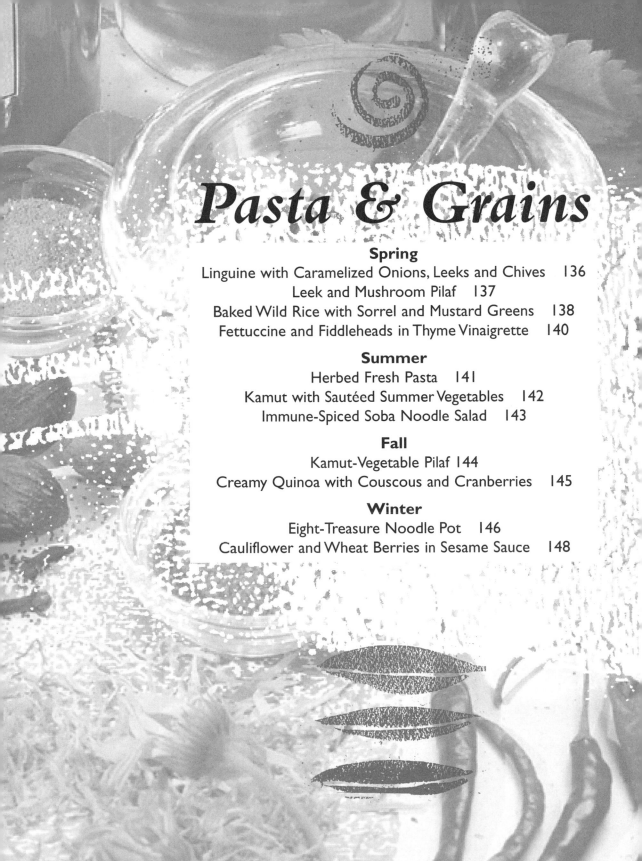

Pasta & Grains

Linguine with Caramelized Onions, Leeks and Chives

Serves 4 to 6

TIP

Slow cooking or roasting brings out the sugars in allium vegetables.

VARIATIONS

Substitute: 1 tbsp (15 mL) white vinegar for wine and increase stock by 1/2 cup (125 mL).

3 tbsp	olive oil	45 mL
4	large red or yellow onions, quartered and thinly sliced	4
2 cups	sliced leeks (wild or domestic)	500 mL
1	bay leaf	1
1 tbsp	chopped fresh rosemary	15 mL
2	cloves garlic, minced	2
1/2 cup	healing white wine (see pages 44–45)	125 mL
1 cup	stock	250 mL
1/4 cup	chopped fresh chives	50 mL
12 oz	linguine	375 g

1. In a large skillet, heat oil over medium-high heat. Stir in onions and leeks; cook for about 3 minutes. Reduce heat to low; add bay leaf and rosemary. Cook, stirring often, for 8 to 12 minutes or until onions are golden brown and soft.

2. Add garlic and wine; cook for 5 minutes or until wine is reduced by half. Add stock; cook for 15 to 20 minutes or until liquid is reduced by a third. Stir in chives.

3. Meanwhile, in a large pot of boiling water, cook linguine for 6 to 8 minutes or until tender but firm. Drain pasta and toss with sauce. Season to taste with salt and pepper if desired.

Leek and Mushroom Pilaf

TIP

Short-grain Italian arborio rice works best for this recipe. (Brown rice does not take up the stock in the same way.)

VARIATIONS

Substitute: Fresh morells, other wild mushrooms or maitake mushrooms for shiitake mushrooms.

Preheat oven to 375° F (190° C) Small baking dish		
1	head garlic	1
2 tsp	olive oil	10 mL
2 tbsp	butter	25 mL
1 cup	chopped wild or domestic leeks	250 mL
2 cups	coarsely chopped shiitake mushrooms	500 mL
3 tbsp	fresh thyme leaves	45 mL
1 cup	arborio rice	250 mL
1/4 cup	healing wine (see pages 44–45)	50 mL
3+ cups	stock	750 mL
1/2 cup	freshly grated Parmesan cheese	125 mL

1. Slice 1/4 inch (1 cm) off top of garlic, leaving skins on. Place garlic cut-side up; in baking dish; drizzle with oil. Cover dish with lid or foil; bake in preheated oven for 35 to 40 minutes or until golden and cloves are very soft. Remove from oven and allow to cool.

2. In a large skillet, heat butter over medium–high heat. Add leeks and mushrooms; cook for 5 minutes or until soft. Stir in thyme and rice. Cook for another 3 minutes, stirring constantly.

3. Stir in wine; squeeze roasted garlic into rice mixture; cook for 2 minutes. Add stock and bring to a boil. Reduce heat to medium; cook, stirring, for 20 minutes or until rice is tender and mixture is creamy. Add more stock if pilaf is dry. The rice should be tender but firm and moist.

4. Remove from heat; stir in Parmesan cheese. Season to taste with salt and pepper.

Baked Wild Rice with Sorrel and Mustard Greens

Serves 6

Preheat oven to 350° F (180° C) 6-cup (1.5 L) casserole, greased		
1 1/2 cups	stock	375 mL
1/2 cup	brown rice	125 mL
1/2 cup	wild rice	125 mL
1	egg	1
1 cup	plain yogurt	250 mL
1/4 cup	basil or herb pesto	50 mL
1 cup	torn sorrel	250 mL
1 cup	torn mustard greens	250 mL
1/2 cup	sunflower seeds	125 mL

1. In a large pot over medium-high heat, bring stock to a boil. Add brown and wild rice; cover, reduce heat and simmer for 30 minutes. Cool rice slightly.

2. In a large bowl, beat egg. Whisk in yogurt and pesto. Add sorrel, mustard greens and sunflower seeds; mix well.

3. Stir cooled rice into yogurt mixture. Season to taste with salt and pepper if desired. Transfer to prepared dish; bake in preheated oven for 20 to 30 minutes or until heated through.

WILD RICE (MANOMIN)

For more than 1000 years, Ojibway and other first peoples have harvested manomin in mid- to late August. "Manomin" is from Manitou, meaning "Great Spirit" and mee-nun, meaning "delicacy".

Gleaned from the brown and green reeds of the long-stemmed annual plant (Zizania palustris) that grows primarily in the shallow waters of northern Ontario, Manitoba and Minnesota, wild rice is a sacred plant. It is central to the Ojibway religion and the foundation of their belief system. At the same time, it was a staple food, one that could be stored for years against times of famine. Always taken in reverence and with a prayer of thanksgiving, manomin is actually not a rice but a member of the grass family, like corn. Unique to North America, it is now not even wild, as the native hunting and fishing societies have sowed new strands of it throughout their territory for centuries (seasonal camps were established as early as 800 A.D. near the dense, marshy stands of wild rice).

Early explorers and Jesuits learned about manomin from the first peoples and used it for survival, according to early historical records.

The ripe grain is harvested by traditional methods used for hundreds of years. The rice pickers paddle canoes through passages in the rice stands, parallel to the shore, and tip the stalks over the boat. The green, mature grain is thrashed directly into the canoe using a cedar stick. It takes about 5 to 10 minutes to pick 1 lb (500 g) of wild rice by hand and skilled ricers can get up to 500 lbs (250 kg) of raw rice in a day.

Traditional processing involves three steps: sun-drying green rice to prevent mildew or fermentation; parching over a fire to loosen the husks; and separating the grain from the husk. Cleaning, separating by length and grading is done by hand. It takes about 2 1/2 lbs (1.25 kg) of green rice to make 1 lb (500 g) of processed wild rice.

Wild rice has more protein than wheat and brown or white rice, less fat than corn and is high in thiamine, riboflavin, niacin and potassium. Use wild rice in recipes where brown or white rice is called for, reducing the amount of raw wild rice by about one-third because wild rice cooks up more than regular rice. Use the whole, cooked grain in soups, salads, breads and cakes and as a breakfast cereal.

To cook wild rice: In a medium saucepan, bring 2 cups (500 mL) water to a boil. Add 1 cup (250 mL) wild rice, cover and adjust heat to keep water just under a boil. Simmer about 40 minutes or until rice is tender and most of the water is absorbed. Drain if necessary. Makes about 3 cups (750 mL) cooked wild rice.

Fettuccine and Fiddleheads in Thyme Vinaigrette

Serves 4

TIP

In early spring the ostrich fern pushes its tightly wound, round shoots through the mulch along streams and riverbanks. First-time gatherers should go with experienced foragers in order to correctly identify the fiddlehead stalks.

VARIATIONS

Substitute: Snow peas or asparagus for fiddleheads; Bean sprouts for rhubarb.

4 cups	water	1 L
2 cups	fresh fiddleheads, washed and trimmed	500 mL
12 oz	fettuccine noodles	375 g
2 tbsp	olive oil	25 mL
1/2 cup	chopped red onions	125 mL
1/2 cup	chopped rhubarb	125 mL
2 tbsp	soya sauce	25 mL
1 tbsp	sesame oil	15 mL
1 tbsp	maple syrup	15 mL
2 tbsp	fresh thyme leaves	25 mL

1. In a large pot over medium–high heat, bring water to a boil. Add fiddleheads, bring back to a boil and cook for 2 minutes. Remove fiddleheads with a slotted spoon to drain; keep water boiling.

2. Add noodles to boiling fiddlehead water. Cover, reduce heat and simmer for 6 to 10 minutes or until just tender. Drain.

3. Meanwhile, in a large wok or skillet, heat oil over medium heat. Cook onion for 5 minutes or until soft. Stir in rhubarb; cook, stirring, for another 5 minutes. Drizzle soya sauce, sesame oil and maple syrup over onion mixture. Stir in fiddleheads and thyme leaves. Cook, stirring, for 1 minute. Toss with cooked noodles and serve.

Herbed Fresh Pasta

Serves 4

TIP

For a zippy change, try a hot salsa instead of the pesto.

VARIATIONS

Substitute: Red wine vinegar for healing wine; hot tomato salsa for pesto; Any pesto for basil pesto.

1 tbsp	butter	15 mL
1 tbsp	olive oil	15 mL
3 cups	sliced red or Spanish onions	750 mL
1/4 cup	healing wine (see pages 44–45)	50 mL
2 tbsp	candied ginger root *or* burdock root, finely chopped	25 mL
1/4 cup	basil pesto	50 mL
12 oz	fresh whole wheat pasta	375 g

1. In a large pan, heat butter and oil over medium heat. Add onions; cook, stirring, for 5 minutes.

2. Add wine and ginger. Reduce heat to medium–low; cook onions for 10 to 15 minutes or until caramelized. Remove from heat, stir in pesto. Season to taste with salt and pepper if desired.

3. Meanwhile, in a large pot, bring water to a boil. Stir in pasta; cook for 3 to 5 minutes if fresh, 8 to 10 minutes if dried, or until tender but firm. Drain. Toss with onion mixture and serve.

RHUBARB (RHEUM RHAPONTICUM)

Rhubarb, a member of the Polygonaceae family, is actually a vegetable although it is generally used in cooking as a fruit. It is a hardy perennial that thrives in areas having cold winters and hot summers and prefers dry soil. Harvested in spring and early summer, only rhubarb stalks are safe for human consumption; the leaves contain toxic amounts of oxalic acid.

Rhubarb originated in southern Siberia, the Himalayas and east Asia. Its name combines the Greek Rha, *with the Latin word,* barbarium *giving some indication as to what the ancients thought of those who first picked and ate it. The Chinese first recorded medicinal astringent and purgative qualities of rhubarb's roots — around 2700 B.C. Europeans are known to have used it medicinally in the 17th century, but it was not*

until the late 18th century that it came into common use as a food. The Victorians popularized the use of rhubarb as a fruit after discoveries that it could be "forced" to grow in greenhouses, thus providing a fresh fruit for the table at a time of year when real fruit was scarce. By the mid-1800s, it had been well established as a pie fruit (actually being called "pie plant") in the United States.

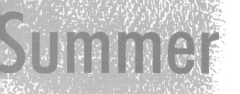

Summer

Kamut with Sautéed Summer Vegetables

Serves 6 to 8

TIP

Soaking kamut overnight reduces the cooking time.

VARIATIONS

Substitute: Any cooked whole grain for kamut.

1 1/4 cups	kamut	300 mL
1 1/2 cups	stock	375 mL
2 tbsp	olive oil	25 mL
1 cup	chopped red bell peppers	250 mL
1 cup	coarsely chopped zucchini	250 mL
1 cup	fresh corn kernels	250 mL
1 cup	peas	250 mL
1/4 cup	chopped fresh parsley	50 mL
1 tbsp	soya sauce	15 mL

1. In a medium bowl, combine kamut and stock. Cover and refrigerate for at least 4 hours or overnight.

2. The next day, in a medium saucepan, bring stock and kamut to a boil. Reduce heat and simmer for 45 to 60 minutes or until kamut is tender and most of liquid is absorbed. Drain, cool in a large colander.

3. In a medium skillet, heat oil over medium-high heat. Add red peppers, zucchini, corn and peas. Cook for 3 to 4 minutes or until vegetables are tender-crisp.

4. Stir in cooked kamut, parsley and soya sauce. Serve warm or chilled.

Immune-Spiced Soba Noodle Salad

Serves 4

TIP

Soba noodles are straight brown buck-wheat flour noodles popular in Japan. They have a nutty flavor some-what like whole wheat and are best served at room temperature or cold — which makes this a great picnic dish. Look for North American soba noodles in health food/alternative stores or some supermarkets. Imported brands can be found in Japanese markets.

VARIATIONS

Substitute: Chinese egg noodles or other whole grains for soba noodles; Peanut butter for cashew butter; Olive oil for sesame oil; Regular vine-gar for rice vinegar; 1 tbsp (15 mL) maple syrup or molasses for echinacea root in syrup.

8 oz	soba noodles	250 g
3 tbsp	cashew butter	45 mL
2 tbsp	chopped candied echinacea root in syrup	25 mL
2 tbsp	soya sauce	25 mL
1 tbsp	roasted sesame oil	15 mL
1	clove garlic, minced	1
2 tbsp	minced ginger root	25 mL
1 tbsp	rice vinegar	15 mL
1	dried hot red chili pepper, crushed (or to taste)	1
1/4 cup	chopped fresh parsley	50 mL

1. In a pot of boiling water over medium-high heat, cook noodles until just tender; drain. Rinse under cold water; drain well.

2. Meanwhile, in a food processor, blender or morter with pestle, purée cashew butter, echinacea, soya sauce, sesame oil, garlic, ginger root, rice vinegar and chili pepper. Season to taste with salt and pepper, if desired. Toss with noodles, add parsley. Serve at room tempera-ture or chilled. Keeps for up to 3 days in refrigerator.

Kamut-Vegetable Pilaf

Serves 6

TIP

To soak kamut or spelt properly, place in a large bowl and cover with water. Allow to sit in the refrigerator for at least 4 hours or overnight.

VARIATIONS

Substitute: Shiitake mushrooms (or any other wild mushroom) for portobello mushrooms.

6 1/2 cups	stock	1.75 L
1 3/4 cups	soaked kamut *or* spelt kernels	425 mL
1 cup	healing wine (see pages 44-45)	250 mL
1 tbsp	olive oil	15 mL
2 cups	sliced portobello mushrooms	500 mL
1	onion, chopped	1
1	clove garlic, minced	1
2 cups	diced sweet potatoes *or* turnips	500 mL
2 cups	small Brussels sprouts	500 mL
2 tsp	dried thyme	10 mL
2 tsp	dried sage	10 mL
1/2 cup	freshly grated Parmesan cheese	125 mL

1. In a large, heavy skillet over medium-high heat, combine 3 1/2 cups (875 mL) stock with kamut kernels. Bring to a boil; reduce heat and simmer, stirring occasionally, for 25 minutes or until liquid is absorbed and kernels are tender. Stir in wine.

2. Meanwhile, in a large saucepan, heat oil over medium-high heat. Add mushrooms, onion and garlic; cook, stirring, over medium heat for 5 minutes or until mushrooms are softened. Stir in remaining stock, sweet potatoes, Brussels sprouts, thyme and sage. Bring to a boil; reduce heat and simmer, stirring occasionally, for 8 to 10 minutes or until vegetables are tender.

3. Stir kernels into vegetable mixture and heat through. Sprinkle with cheese; season to taste with salt and pepper if desired.

Creamy Quinoa with Couscous and Cranberries

Makes 3 cups (750 mL)

1 cup	wholewheat couscous	250 mL
1/4 cup	almonds	50 mL
1/2 cup	quinoa, thoroughly rinsed	125 mL
2 1/2 cups	water	625 mL
1	can (14 oz [398 mL]) coconut milk	1
1/2 cup	dried cranberries	125 mL
1/2 tsp	cinnamon	2 mL
1 tsp	ground licorice	5 mL

TIP

Couscous is not a whole grain but a product made from semolina flour — rolled, steamed and easy to cook. It is teamed here with quinoa for extra nutrients. Serve as a warm breakfast cereal, a sweet-tart accompaniment to steamed vegetables, or as a satisfying dessert.

Look for ground licorice in health food stores.

Quinoa has a bitter taste unless well rinsed.

VARIATIONS

Substitute: Soy milk for coconut milk; Dried cherries or raisins for cranberries.

1. In a food processor or blender, grind 1/2 cup (125 mL) couscous with almonds to a fine powder. Set aside.

2. In a medium-sized saucepan over medium-high heat, bring quinoa and water to a boil. Reduce heat to medium-low; cover and cook for 10 minutes. Stir in remaining couscous; replace cover and cook for 5 to 8 minutes or until liquid is absorbed and quinoa looks transparent.

3. Stir in ground couscous mixture, coconut milk, cranberries, cinnamon and licorice. Bring to a boil; cook, uncovered, for 2 minutes or until mixture thickens.

4. Remove from heat; cover pan and set aside for 5 minutes. Serve warm.

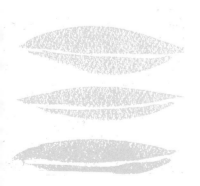

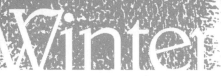

Eight-Treasure Noodle Pot

TIP

Traditionally, fish, shrimp and scallops are three of the treasures in this dish. If desired, in step 2, add 8 oz (250 g) each of firm fish (such as cod, haddock or whitefish), shrimp in the shell (rinsed and drained), and fresh scallops. Increase the stock by 1 1/2 cups (375 mL).

VARIATIONS

Substitute: Regular green cabbage for Chinese cabbage; 1 cup (250 mL) small whole shiitake mushrooms in step 2 for dried black mushrooms; 12 oz (375 g) Chinese egg noodles (do not pre-soak) for cellophane noodles.

Omit: Ginseng and astragalus, if not available.

2	dried black mushrooms	2
1 oz	cellophane noodles (bean threads)	25 g
2 tbsp	olive oil	25 mL
2	cloves garlic, minced	2
1 tbsp	chopped ginger root	15 mL
2 cups	Chinese cabbage, cored and shredded	500 mL
2 cups	broccoli florets	500 mL
4 cups	stock	1 L
1 tbsp	powdered ginseng root	15 mL
2	pieces dried astragalus	2

1. In a mixing bowl, cover mushrooms with boiling water. Set aside. In another mixing bowl, cover noodles with hot tap water to soften. Set aside.

2. Meanwhile, in a large Dutch oven, heat oil over medium heat. Stir in garlic, ginger, Chinese cabbage and broccoli. Cook, stirring, for 2 to 3 minutes. Do not brown.

3. Stir in stock and astragalus. Bring to a boil; reduce heat and simmer 20 minutes or until vegetables are tender-crisp.

4. Drain mushrooms; slice. Drain noodles. Add to mixture with ginseng. Remove and discard astragalus before serving.

ASIAN NOODLES

To the Chinese, noodles are a symbol of longevity — the longer the noodles, the longer the life, especially if served on birthdays. For this reason, Chinese cooks never cut noodles.

Asian noodles are available at Asian/Oriental markets, some specialty food shops, alternative/health stores and some urban supermarkets.

Rice noodles: *Made from rice flour, off-white rice noodles vary in width from thick to thin and in shape, round or flat. The most popular are thin, known as rice sticks or vermicelli. Delicate in flavor, rice noodles are usually softened in water for 15 to 30 minutes before using and turn a brighter white when cooked.*

Wheat-flour noodles: *Can be made with or without egg, the difference being slight, both in taste and nutrients. Usually flat, wheat-flour noodles are sold dried or fresh and sometimes frozen. Japanese udon are fat, white and slippery when fresh. Japanese ramen are thin egg noodles used in Oriental-style instant soups (Chinese* dan mian *are the Chinese equivalent).*

Cellophane noodles: *These fine silvery filaments are also called "bean threads" because they are made from the protein-rich mung bean. The noodles are soaked in hot water before using. They are slippery, become almost clear upon cooking, and soak up the tastes of marinades, dressings and stir-fry ingredients.*

Buckwheat-flour noodles: *Also known as soba, these Japanese noodles are often made with some wheat flour as well as buckwheat. Long, perfectly straight, usually square, they are best served cold with a spiced dipping sauce or dressing along with lightly steamed vegetables.*

Potato-starch noodles: *Korean* dang myun *noodles are transparent and slippery, made from the combined starch of the regular and sweet potato. Soak briefly in hot water before use.*

Cauliflower and Wheat Berries in Sesame Sauce

Serves 4 to 6

Tahini

Tahini is a paste made by grinding sesame seeds. It is used for flavor and as a thickener in sauces, dips and soups.

To make tahini: *In a blender, grind 2 tbsp (25 mL) sesame seeds until smooth. Add 1/2 tsp (2 mL) sesame oil and 1/4 cup (50 mL) tepid water. Blend until smooth. Makes about 1/2 cup (125 mL).*

1	head cauliflower, separated into florets	1
1 1/2 cups	wheat berries	375 mL
1/4 cup	olive oil	50 mL
3 tbsp	rice vinegar	45 mL
2 tbsp	sesame oil	25 mL
2 tbsp	soya sauce	25 mL
1 tbsp	tahini	15 mL
2	cloves garlic, minced	2
1 cup	green onions, diagonally sliced	250 mL
3 tbsp	sesame seeds	45 mL

1. In a large pot of boiling water over medium-high heat, cook cauliflower for 5 to 7 minutes or until just tender-crisp. Using tongs, transfer cauliflower to colander; rinse with cold water. Drain.

2. To the same pot of boiling water, add wheat berries; gently boil, uncovered, for 1 hour or until tender. Drain and allow to cool.

3. Meanwhile, in a medium bowl, whisk together olive oil, vinegar, sesame oil, soya sauce, tahini and garlic.

4. In a large serving bowl, combine cauliflower, wheat berries and green onions. Drizzle with sesame sauce; toss gently to coat well. Sprinkle with sesame seeds.

SESAME SEEDS (SESAMUM INDICUM)

A tall plant with a single stalk, native to India. It is also grown in Africa, Afghanistan, and Indonesia. Seeds of the herb are sold in a variety of ways: whole (with the hulls), raw (dark); hulled and polished, raw (white); and hulled and roasted (tan). Sesame seeds are a good source of incomplete protein, which works well with legumes or whole grains, and lend a nutty taste to dishes.

Sesame oil pressed from raw seeds is clear and golden and is used in cooking, cosmetics and as a solvent in medicinal remedies. When pressed from roasted seeds, the oil is dark amber and imparts a rich, roasted flavor to foods. Sesame seed oil (often called "benne" oil after the African word for sesame), is exceptionally stable and is a source of vitamin E, an antioxidant.

Actions: *emollient, laxative.*

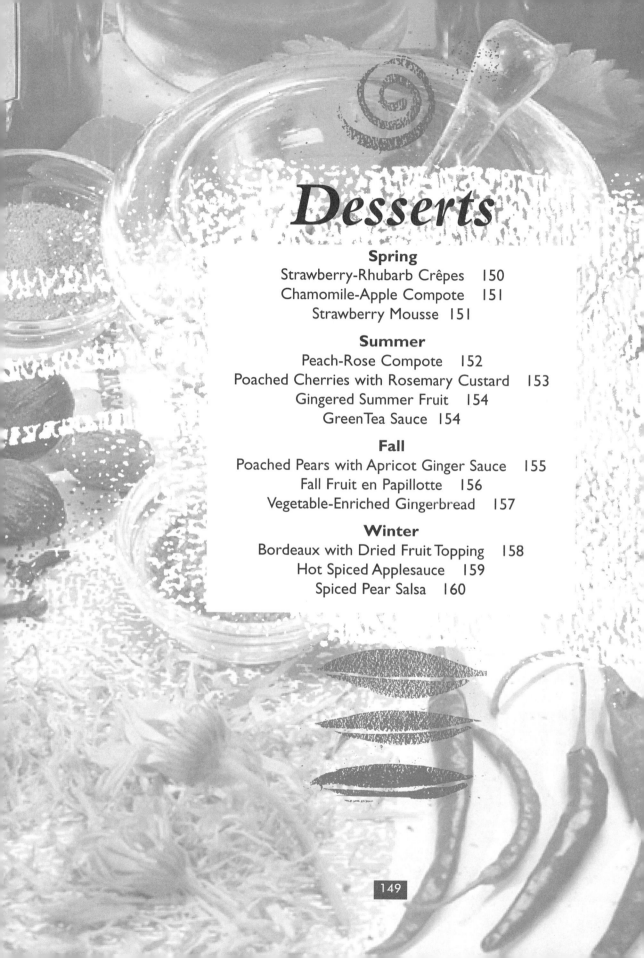

Desserts

Spring
Strawberry-Rhubarb Crêpes   150
Chamomile-Apple Compote   151
Strawberry Mousse   151

Summer
Peach-Rose Compote   152
Poached Cherries with Rosemary Custard   153
Gingered Summer Fruit   154
Green Tea Sauce   154

Fall
Poached Pears with Apricot Ginger Sauce   155
Fall Fruit en Papillotte   156
Vegetable-Enriched Gingerbread   157

Winter
Bordeaux with Dried Fruit Topping   158
Hot Spiced Applesauce   159
Spiced Pear Salsa   160

Strawberry-Rhubarb Crêpes

1 cup	yogurt	250 mL
1/2 cup	whole wheat flour	125 mL
2	eggs	2
3/4 cup	soy milk	175 mL
2 tbsp	melted butter	25 mL
1 cup	chopped rhubarb	250 mL
1/4 cup	orange juice	50 mL
2 tbsp	brown rice syrup	25 mL
1 cup	sliced strawberries	250 mL

1. In a sieve lined with cheesecloth and set over a bowl, drain yogurt for at least 3 hours in refrigerator.

2. Place flour in a large bowl. In a small bowl, whisk egg with milk and butter. Gradually whisk into flour until a thin batter forms. Allow to sit for about 30 minutes.

3. Lightly oil a medium skillet; heat over medium-high heat. Pour in about 3 tbsp (45 mL) batter; tilt pan so batter covers bottom with a thin film. Cook for 45 seconds or until crêpe is brown on bottom. Flip and brown other side for about 15 seconds. Lightly oil skillet before cooking each crêpe. Allow to cool before stacking.

4. In a medium saucepan over medium-low heat, combine rhubarb and orange juice. Simmer, covered, for 3 minutes or until liquid is released. Remove cover and cook 7 minutes or until rhubarb is soft. Remove from heat; stir in rice syrup. Cool.

5. In a medium bowl, mix together cooled rhubarb, strawberries and drained yogurt. Refrigerate until ready to use.

6. Spread 2 rounded tbsp (45 mL) filling over center of each crêpe. Fold each crepe in half, then in half again, to create a wedge shape. Serve at room temperature.

Chamomile-Apple Compote

Serves 4

TIP

Garnish with fresh whipped cream or yogurt cheese (see step 1 in facing recipe for technique).

VARIATIONS

Substitute: Maple syrup or brown rice syrup for ginger syrup; Burdock root or other candied root for ginger.

6	apples, cored and cut into slices	6
1/4 cup	chopped raisins	50 mL
1/4 cup	applesauce	50 mL
1/4 cup	apple juice	50 mL
2 tbsp	finely chopped candied ginger	25 mL
2 tbsp	ginger syrup	25 mL
1/4 cup	fresh chamomile flowers	50 mL
1 tbsp	agar agar flakes	15 mL

1. In a large pot, combine apples, raisins, applesauce and juice. Cover and cook over medium heat, stirring occasionally, for 10 minutes. Add ginger, syrup, chamomile and agar agar. Simmer for another 15 minutes or until apples are tender. Serve warm or at room temperature.

Strawberry Mousse

Serves 4

TIP

Use each fresh fruit or berry as they come into season for this light dessert.

VARIATIONS

Substitute: Basil for sweet cicely.

2 cups	soy milk	500 mL
2 tbsp	agar agar flakes	25 mL
2 tbsp	fresh sweet cicely, finely chopped	25 mL
2 cups	hulled strawberries	500 mL
1 tbsp	brown rice syrup	15 mL

1. In a medium saucepan over medium heat, bring soy milk to a gentle simmer. Stir in agar agar and sweet cicely. Reduce heat; simmer slowly for 5 minutes, stirring occasionally.

2. In a blender, combine strawberries, rice syrup and soy milk; blend until smooth.

3. Pour mousse into a serving bowl or individual dishes. Chill for 2 hours or until set. Garnish with whole strawberries or sweet cicely leaves.

Peach-Rose Compote

Makes 5 cups (1.25 L)

TIP

Serve chilled as you would jam or hot over porridge.

VARIATIONS

Substitute: Water or orange water for rosewater.

6	peaches, peeled and coarsely chopped	6
2 cups	pitted fresh apricots, quartered	500 mL
1/4 cup	rosewater	50 mL
2 tbsp	ginger syrup	25 mL
1/2 cup	fresh rose petals	125 mL

1. In a large saucepan over medium heat, combine peaches, apricots, rosewater and ginger syrup. Cover, bring to a simmer, then reduce heat. Gently simmer for 15 minutes or until apricots are soft. Stir in rose petals.

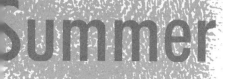

Poached Cherries with Rosemary Custard

Serves 4

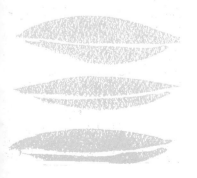

TIP

Infusing the milk as it heats imparts not only the flavor of the herbs but their medicinal benefits as well. Keep a lid on the milk as it scalds and while it is cooling in step 1. For a lighter custard, beat 2 egg whites until glossy, sprinkle with 1 tbsp (15 mL) sugar and continue to beat until stiff but not dry. Fold into custard in step 2.

VARIATIONS

Substitute: Cinnamon for licorice; Tarragon for rosemary.

4 cups	pitted whole cherries	1 L
3/4 cup	apple juice	175 mL
1/2 cup	red wine	125 mL
1/2 cup	soy milk	125 mL
1	3-inch (7.5 cm) vanilla bean	1
1	2-inch (5 cm) licorice root	1
1	rosemary sprig	1
12 oz	firm "silken style" tofu	375 g

1. In a medium saucepan, combine cherries, apple juice and wine; bring to a boil. Reduce heat, and simmer gently for 10 minutes or until cherries are just tender.

2. In a small saucepan over medium–low heat, combine soy milk, vanilla bean, licorice and rosemary. Cover and lightly simmer until bubbles form around outside of pan. Remove from heat and allow to cool with lid on. Strain and discard vanilla, licorice and rosemary.

3. In a food processor or blender, process tofu for 30 seconds or until smooth. With motor running, add cooled herbed milk through funnel. Process until blended and smooth.

4. To serve, spoon warm cherries into bowls; top with custard. Keep custard in refrigerator, covered, for 1 to 2 days.

Summer

Gingered Summer Fruit

**Makes 2 1/2 cups
(625 mL)**

TIP

Use nectarines, peaches, plums, cherries, gooseberries, elderberries, or currants for this easy summer sauce. Serve with frozen yogurt, tofu cheesecake and other desserts.

VARIATIONS

Substitute: 2 tsp (10 mL) cornstarch for agar agar (mix with lemon juice before adding to fruit in step 1); Maple syrup for burdock syrup.

1 lb	fruit, pitted (cut larger fruit into quarters; smaller fruit into halves)	500 g
1/4 cup	*burdock syrup* (see page 39 for technique) *or* ginger or dandelion syrup	50 mL
2 tsp	minced ginger root	10 mL
2 tbsp	fresh lemon juice	25 mL
1 tbsp	agar agar flakes	15 mL

1. In a saucepan over medium heat, combine fruit, burdock and ginger. Cover; cook for 5 minutes or until juices release and fruit is slightly tender.

2. Stir in lemon juice and agar agar. Cook, stirring, for 2 minutes or until agar melts. Serve warm or cold (mixture will thicken when cooled).

Green Tea Sauce

**Makes about
1 1/2 cups (375 mL)**

TIP

This tart sauce is excellent with grilled chicken or to top off a dessert; sweeten with up to 2 tbsp (25 mL) honey, if desired.

VARIATIONS

Substitute: Any herbal tea bag for raspberry; Raisins for apricots.

2 tbsp	green tea leaves	25 mL
2 cups	boiling water	500 mL
2	raspberry herbal tea bags	2
1/4 cup	dried cherries	50 mL
1/4 cup	chopped dried apricots	50 mL
1/2 cup	apple juice or apple cider	125 mL
1 tbsp	finely chopped ginger root	15 mL

1. Tie green tea leaves in a cheesecloth square or place in a tea ball. In a non-reactive medium saucepan, pour boiling water over green tea, raspberry tea and dried cherries. Cover and steep for 15 minutes. Remove green tea and tea bags, pressing gently to extract all liquid.

2. Stir in apricots, apple juice and ginger. Cover and bring tea to a boil over medium–high heat. Adjust heat to keep liquid at a gentle boil; cook for 20 minutes or until reduced to 1 1/2 cups (375 mL).

3. Remove 1 cup (250 mL) of sauce; purée in a food processor. Combine with remaining sauce. Serve warm or cold.

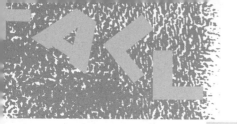

Poached Pears with Apricot Ginger Sauce

TIP

Apples or plums also work well in this fall dessert.

VARIATIONS

Substitute: 1/2 inch (1 cm) fresh minced ginger root or 1 tsp (5 mL) ground ginger for candied ginger; 1/4 cup (50 mL) chopped walnuts for candied burdock.

2 cups	apple juice	500 mL
Half	vanilla bean	Half
1	3-inch (7.5 cm) licorice root	1
1	sprig fresh tarragon	1
4	pears, sliced in half	4
1/3 cup	finely chopped dried apricots	75 mL
1 tbsp	finely chopped candied ginger	15 mL
3 tbsp	chopped candied burdock	45 mL
1 cup	plain yogurt	250 mL

1. In a large skillet over medium heat, combine apple juice, vanilla bean, licorice and tarragon. Add pears, cut-side down. Reduce heat and simmer gently for 8 minutes or until pears are tender. Remove pears with slotted spoon, set aside.

2. Remove and discard vanilla bean, licorice and tarragon. Add apricots and ginger; bring to a boil. Reduce heat and simmer, stirring occasionally, for 15 to 20 minutes or until mixture is syrupy.

3. Remove and discard core from pear halves. Arrange pears on individual plates; spoon apricot sauce over. Garnish with chopped burdock and yogurt. Serve warm.

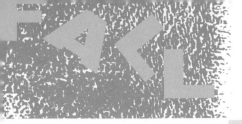

Fall Fruit en Papillotte

Preheat oven to 350° F (180° C)
4 sheets parchment paper, 12 by 18 inches (30 by 40 cm)
Baking sheet

1/4 cup	raisins	50mL
1/4 cup	chopped pecans	50mL
1/4 cup	chopped candied ginger	50mL
4	1-inch (2.5 cm) pieces cinnamon stick	4
4	1-inch (2.5 cm) pieces licorice root	4
4	1-inch (2.5 cm) pieces vanilla bean	4
4	whole cloves	4
1	pear, cored and cut into eighths	1
1	apple, cored and cut into eighths	1
4	dried or fresh apricots, halved	4
1	peach, cored and quartered	1
1	plum, cored and quartered	1
1/2 cup	apple cider	125 mL
1 tsp	butter	5 mL

1. Fold each sheet of parchment paper in half. Trim to make 4 heart-shaped pieces.

2. Open each heart of parchment paper. On one side of fold line add 1 tbsp (15 mL) each raisins, pecans and ginger; 1 each cinnamon stick, licorice root, vanilla bean and clove; 2 each pear, apple and apricot pieces; 1 each peach and plum quarters. Sprinkle 2 tbsp (25 mL) cider over each; top with 1/4 tsp (1 mL) butter.

3. Fold other half of parchment heart over fruit. Beginning at curve of heart, roll cut ends together to seal.

4. Place fruit packages on baking sheet. Bake in preheated oven for 30 to 40 minutes or until apples and pears are tender. Slide each package onto a serving plate; cut an "X" on top of each package with a knife. Pull back tips of "X" to make an opening. Serve warm in parchment.

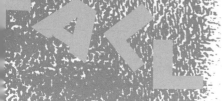

Vegetable-Enriched Gingerbread

Serves 8 to 12

TIP

Children love the bright red spots in this bread — especially if you are a bit vague about exactly what they are. Even with the small amount of sugar, this is one "cake" or sweet bread that I let my daughter have for breakfast, at snacks and just about any other time the hungry bunnies strike.

Preheat oven to 350° F (180° C)
9-inch (22.5 cm) square baking pan, greased

1/2 cup	butter	125 mL
1/2 cup	granulated sugar	125 mL
2	eggs	2
1/3 cup	molasses	75 mL
1/2 cup	plain yogurt	125 mL
1 tsp	vanilla extract	5 mL
2 cups	whole wheat flour	500 mL
1 tbsp	baking powder	15 mL
1 tbsp	ground cinnamon	15 mL
1/2 tsp	salt	2 mL
1/4 tsp	ground nutmeg	1 mL
1/4 tsp	ground allspice	1 mL
1/4 tsp	ground cloves	1 mL
2/3 cup	grated carrots	150 mL
2/3 cup	grated parsnips	150 mL
1 cup	grated beets	250 mL
1	1-inch (2.5 cm) candied ginger square, minced	1

1. In a large bowl, cream butter. Beat in sugar until light and fluffy. Beat in eggs, one at a time, then molasses, yogurt and vanilla.

2. Sift together flour, baking powder, cinnamon, salt, nutmeg, allspice and cloves; beat into butter mixture. Stir in carrots, parsnips, beets and ginger. Batter will be thick.

3. Transfer batter to prepared pan. Bake in preheated oven for 50 to 60 minutes or until cake springs back when gently pressed in center. Serve with hot applesauce (see recipe, page 159).

Winter

Bordeaux with Dried Fruit Topping

Makes 3 cups (750 mL)

TIP

Use a dry red or white wine — but keep in mind the red will color the other ingredients.

VARIATIONS

Substitute: Healing wine (see pages 44-45) or fruit juice for Bordeaux wine.

Omit: Licorice root if not available.

1/2 cup	orange juice	125 mL
1	4-inch (10 cm) cinnamon stick	1
1	1-inch (2.5 cm) piece ginger root	1
1	1-inch (2.5 cm) piece licorice root	1
1/3 cup	chopped dried dates	75 mL
1/3 cup	chopped apricots	75 mL
1 cup	raisins	250 mL
1 cup	coarsely chopped almonds	250 mL
3 tbsp	brown rice syrup	45 mL
1/2 cup	Bordeaux wine	125 mL
2 cups	plain yogurt	500 mL

1. In a non-reactive saucepan, heat orange juice over medium-high heat. Stir in cinnamon, ginger, licorice, dates, apricots, raisins and almonds. Bring to a boil; cover and reduce heat. Simmer gently for 15 minutes or until fruit is soft.

2. Stir in syrup and wine; heat through. Let cool slightly; remove cinnamon, ginger and licorice root. Spoon over yogurt to serve.

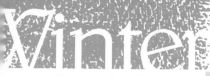

Hot Spiced Applesauce

Serves 4 to 6

TIP

A good dish to serve anyone recovering from the flu.

10	apples, peeled and cut into 1/2-inch (1 cm) slices	10
1 cup	apple cider	250 mL
1 tbsp	apple cider vinegar	15 mL
1 tbsp	butter	15 mL
1 tbsp	rice syrup	15 mL
1 tbsp	finely chopped candied ginger	15 mL
1/2 tsp	cayenne pepper	2 mL
2	crushed whole cloves (or 1/4 tsp [1 mL] ground cloves)	2

1. In a medium saucepan, combine apples, cider, vinegar, butter, rice syrup, ginger and cayenne. Cook, covered, over medium heat for 15 minutes. Uncover; cook 5 more minutes for chunky apple sauce or 15 minutes for smoother sauce, stirring occasionally.

2. Serve hot or chilled with crushed cloves sprinkled over top.

APPLES (MALUS SPP.)

Britain's Crabtree is the native ancestor of all cultivated apple varieties — now numbering over 2,000 and growing in all temperate zones. As early as 1470, Bartholomeus wrote about apples. They were used to treat flu, fevers, gout, eye infections, bronchial complaints, heart problems, lethargy, and anemia. Our wassail bowl or loving cup — a traditional drink for Christmas, weddings and other festive occasions — is a throwback to the ceremony of "wassailing the orchard-trees". Wassail comes from the Anglo Saxon, meaning "to be hale"; the wassailing ritual started with a chant and finished with the farmer tossing a bucket of roasted apples and cider over the trees in his orchard in the hopes that they would bear fruit for many years.

Fresh apples are cleansing for the system, help lower cholesterol, keep blood glucose levels up, and aid digestion; stewed fruit is used for diarrhea and dysentery; the French use the peel in preparations for rheumatism and gout and in urinary tract remedies. Used in cleansing fasts, apples are good sources of vitamin A and also contain vitamins C, B and G (the "appetite vitamin"). Apples are high in two important phytochemicals: pectin, which helps to lower both cholesterol and colon cancer; and boron, thought to help prevent the calcium loss that leads to osteoporosis, boost blood levels of the hormone estrogen (thus assisting menopausal women), and which appears to stimulate the electrical activity of the brain, increasing the ability to perform tasks quickly and efficiently.

Actions: *Tonic, digestive, liver stimulant, diuretic, detoxifying, laxative, antiseptic, lowers cholesterol, anti-rheumatic.*

Winter

Makes 5 cups (1.25 L)

TIP

Use as a dessert topping for yogurt or an accompaniment for vegetable stir-fries or other savory dishes.

VARIATIONS

Substitute: Any juice for pear nectar.

Spiced Pear Salsa

3 tbsp	butter	45 mL
1 cup	chopped onions	250 mL
6	pears, peeled, cored and diced	6
3/4 cup	pear nectar	175 mL
1 tbsp	apple cider vinegar	15 mL
1 tbsp	ground turmeric	15 mL
1 tsp	garam masala	5 mL
1 tsp	ground cardamom	5 mL
1/4 cup	raisins	50 mL
1 tbsp	honey	15 mL

1. In a large saucepan, melt butter over low heat. Stir in onions; cook, stirring occasionally, for 15 minutes or until soft.

2. Stir in pears, nectar, vinegar, turmeric, garam masala, cardamom, raisins and honey. Increase heat and simmer gently for 15 to 30 minutes or until mixture is thick and pears are tender.

FALL FRUIT EN PAPILLOTTE (PAGE 156) ➤

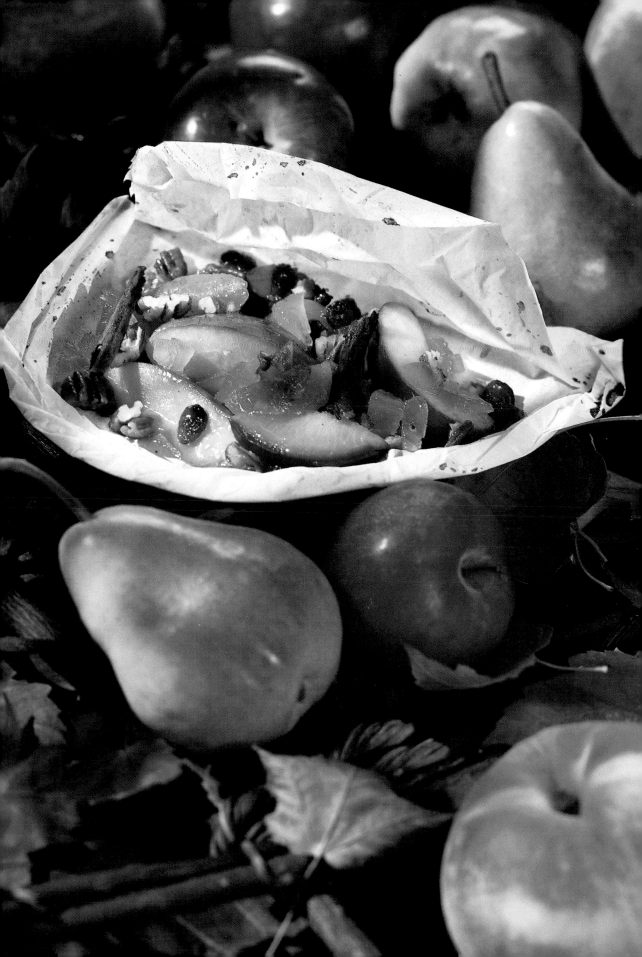

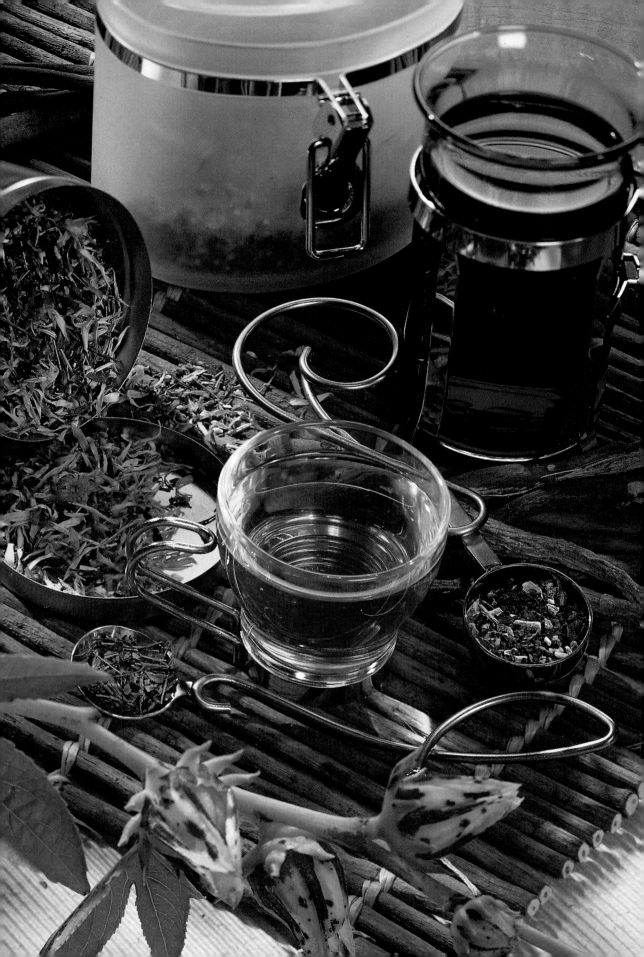

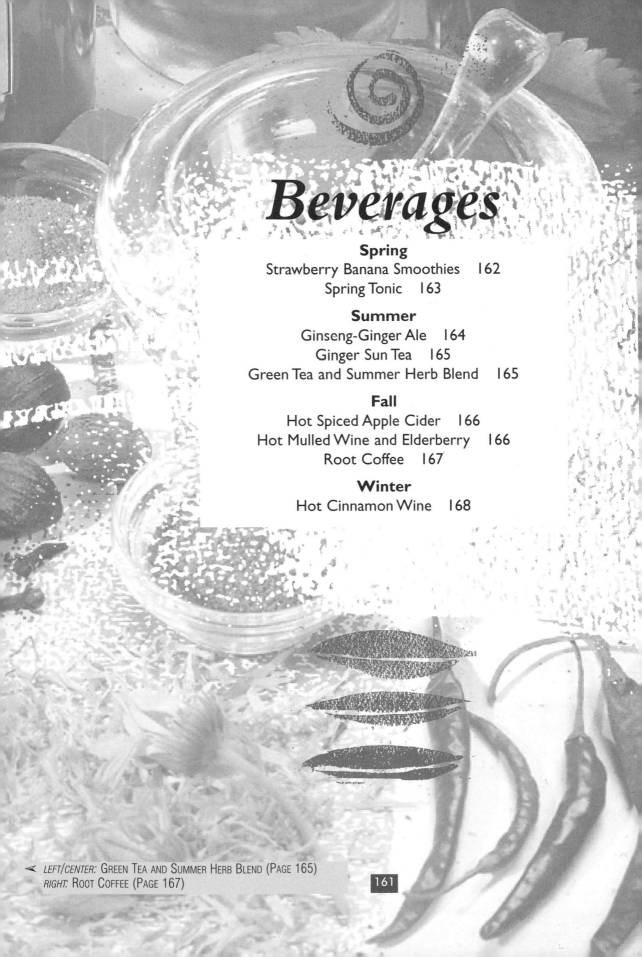

Beverages

◄ *LEFT/CENTER:* GREEN TEA AND SUMMER HERB BLEND (PAGE 165)
RIGHT: ROOT COFFEE (PAGE 167)

Strawberry Banana Smoothies

Makes 4 cups (1 L)

TIP

This refreshing drink can be made in winter using frozen strawberries and reconstituted orange juice.

VARIATIONS

Substitute: Any fresh juice for orange juice.

Add: 1 cup (250 mL) yogurt; 1 tbsp (15 mL) wheat germ; 1 tsp (5 mL) ground ginseng.

1	banana	1
2 cups	fresh strawberries	500 mL
2 cups	fresh orange juice	500 mL

1. Break up banana into a blender or food processor. Turn motor on and add strawberries, then orange juice. Process until smooth.

Spring Tonic

2 cups	water	500 mL
1	fresh ginseng root, chopped	1
1	fresh dandelion root, chopped	1
1	fresh burdock root, chopped	1
2 tbsp	chopped fresh parsley	25 mL
2 tbsp	chopped fresh stinging nettle	25 mL

TIP

One tbsp (15 mL) chopped fresh or dried burdock root gently simmered in 1 cup (250 mL) water for 15 minutes makes a delicious drink on its own. Take 3 or 4 times a day for about a month in the spring.

The addition of alcohol (vodka or gin) acts as a preservative and allows the tonic to be made in larger quantities and stored. Add 1/4 cup (50 mL) alcohol to this recipe, if desired.

VARIATIONS

Add: Honey to taste, if desired.

Dose: 1/2 cup (125 mL), 4 times per day.

1. In a medium saucepan, pour water over ginseng, dandelion and burdock. Cover and bring to a boil over medium heat. Reduce heat and simmer gently for 10 minutes. Remove from heat. Stir in parsley and nettle. Allow to stand, covered, for 20 minutes. Strain into a clean jar, pressing on solids to extract all liquid. Cover and keep in refrigerator for 1 day only.

SPRING TONICS

Spring tonics are an ancient rite of spring that reflect its central theme — self renewal. As recently as the early 1900s, people scurried out for the first tender leaves of such common herbs as dandelion and nettle to concoct these often bitter brews.

By definition, a tonic is an infusion of herbs that invigorates or strengthens the system. Often tonics act as stimulants and alteratives. Taken either hot or cold, tonics restore tone, purify the blood and act as nutritive builders.

Our ancestors knew from time-honored rituals that a few doses of these liquors could put the bite on winter by flushing and reviving even the most sluggish of systems. Recipes were passed on through the generations and by the 1800s, they were showing up in household books.

Grandmother's Family Spring Bitters

"Mandrake root one ounce, dandelion root one ounce, burdock root one ounce, yellow dock root one ounce, prickly ash berries two ounces, marshmallow one ounce, turkey rhubarb half an ounce, gentian one ounce, English camomile flowers one ounce, red clover tops two ounces.

Wash the herbs and roots; put them into an earthen vessel, pour over two quarts of water that has been boiled and cooled; let it stand overnight and soak; in the morning set it on the back of the stove, and steep it five hours; it must not boil, but be nearly ready to boil. Strain it through a cloth, and add half a pint of good gin. Keep it in a cool place. Half a wine-glass taken as a dose twice a day."

from the White House Cook Book, by Hugo Zieman and Mrs. F.L. Gillette, 1887.

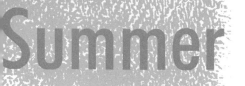
Ginseng-Ginger Ale

Makes 15 cups (3.75 L)

3 cups	water	750 mL
8 oz	fresh ginger root, unpeeled, trimmed and chopped	250 g
1 oz	whole dried ginseng root	25 g
1/2 cup	herbed honey	125 mL
3 tbsp	bruised fresh stevia leaves	45 mL
1/4 cup	bruised fresh peppermint leaves	50 mL
1 tbsp	grated lemon zest	15 mL
1/3 cup	fresh lemon juice	75 mL
12 cups	club soda	3 L
	Fresh peppermint sprigs	

1. In a large non-reactive stock pot, bring water to a boil. Add ginger and ginseng roots; reduce heat and simmer, covered, for 20 minutes.

2. Add honey; stir well to dissolve. Reduce heat to low; add stevia, mint and lemon zest. Cover and heat gently for 10 minutes. Remove pot from heat; allow mixture to stand, covered, for 2 hours or until room temperature.

3. Strain liquid, discarding solids. Stir in lemon juice. Pour into clean or sterilized jars with lids. Store in refrigerator.

4. For each serving, combine 1/4 cup (50 mL) ginseng-ginger ale with 1 cup (250 mL) club soda. Pour over ice in a large glass; garnish with mint sprigs.

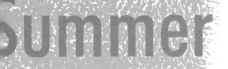

Ginger Sun Tea

Makes 6 cups (1.5 L)

TIP

Sunlight gently warms the water, drawing out the goodness from the herbs.

VARIATIONS

Substitute: 3 teabags for loose green tea; 1 tsp (5 mL) dried stevia leaves for fresh.

	8-cup (2 L) clear glass container	
1	2-inch (5 cm) piece ginger root, unpeeled and thinly sliced	1
4 tbsp	green tea leaves	50 mL
1 tbsp	bruised fresh stevia leaves	15 mL
6 cups	warm water	1.5 L
2 tbsp	ginger syrup	25 mL
	Lemon slices for garnish	

1. In container, combine ginger root, tea leaves, stevia leaves and water. Cover with a lid or clear plastic wrap. Let stand in direct sun, preferably outside, for 3 hours.

2. Strain through a fine sieve into a serving pitcher. Stir in syrup and chill. To serve, fill glasses with ice. Pour in tea and garnish with lemon slice.

Green Tea and Summer Flower Blend

1 part	green tea leaves	1 part
1 part	calendula petals	1 part
1/2 part	St. John's wort petals	1/2 part
1/2 part	echinacea petals	1/2 part
1/4 part	lavender buds	1/4 part

1. Measure and blend all ingredients. Store in a cool, dark, airtight jar.

TIP

Flowers are often nipped back on herb plants to encourage further leaf growth. However, flowers on most edible herbs make a colorful addition to summer dishes and tea blends. Dry herbs and flowers first (see page 36), then measure and blend.

VARIATIONS

Substitute: Any flowering herb petals.

TO MAKE 1 CUP OF TEA

Pour 1 cup (250 mL) boiling water over 1 tsp (15 mL) GREEN TEA AND SUMMER HERB BLEND for mild tea, 2 tsp (10 mL) for stronger tea. Allow to steep 10 minutes; strain and drink while still hot.

Hot Spiced Apple Cider

Makes 8 cups (2 L)

TIP

A warming drink to serve after a chilly fall excursion.

VARIATIONS

Substitute: Elderberry syrup for apple cider vinegar.

8 cups	apple cider	2 L
1	3-inch (7.5 cm) cinnamon stick	1
1	3-inch (7.5 cm) piece vanilla bean	1
3	cloves	3
3	allspice berries	3
1	1-inch (2.5 cm) piece ginger root, unpeeled and grated	1
1 tbsp	dried stevia leaves	15 mL
2 tbsp	honey	25 mL
1 tbsp	apple cider vinegar	15 mL
1 tbsp	butter	15 mL
	Orange or lemon slices	

1. In a large pot, heat apple cider, cinnamon stick, vanilla bean, cloves, allspice berries, ginger root and stevia leaves to just under a boil; simmer for 20 minutes. If desired, strain through a sieve, pressing on solids to extract all liquid. Stir in honey, vinegar and butter until melted. Serve hot with orange or lemon slices.

Hot Mulled Wine and Elderberry

Makes 7 cups (1.75 L)

TIP

Use red or white wine in this recipe. Do not boil wine; simmer just long enough to heat through, then remove from heat.

VARIATIONS

Substitute: Any herb jelly for elderberry.

3 cups	white grape juice	750 mL
1	3-inch (7.5 cm) cinnamon stick	1
1	3-inch (7.5 cm) piece vanilla bean	1
3	cloves	3
3	allspice berries	3
1	1-inch (2.5 cm) piece ginger root, grated	1
1/2 cup	elderberry jelly	125 mL
3 cups	wine	750 mL
	Orange slices	

1. In a saucepan, heat grape juice, cinnamon stick, vanilla bean, cloves, allspice and ginger to just under a boil. Simmer, covered, for 20 minutes. If desired, strain through a sieve, pressing on solids to extract all liquid.
2. Return to pot. Over medium heat, stir in jelly until melted. Add wine; heat through. Serve hot with orange slices for garnish.

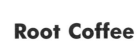

Root Coffee

Makes 2 1/2 cups (625 mL) dried root blend

TIP

There is no resemblance to the taste of coffee with this drink — it has a sweet (especially if the licorice is used) fragrant taste all of its own, and no milk is needed. Use any or all of the roots listed here to blend this rich-tasting coffee substitute. Wait until after the tops of the plants have died back (be sure to note the location of the plants first), but before the ground is frozen, to dig up the roots for this recipe. All of the ingredients — in dried form — are available in alternative/health stores.

VARIATIONS

Roasting the roots lends a richer taste but is not essential.

Substitute: If using dried roots, use 1 cup (250 mL) dried chopped dandelion root, 1 cup (250 mL) dried chopped burdock root and 1/2 cup (125 mL) dried chopped chicory root. Roast at 300° F (150° C) for 20 minutes, stirring once, or until lightly browned. Continue with steps 2 and 3.

Preheat oven to 300° F (150° C) Large baking sheet		
6 to 8	fresh dandelion roots	6 to 8
4 to 6	fresh burdock roots	4 to 6
3 to 4	fresh chicory roots	3 to 4
1	2-inch (5 cm) piece cinnamon stick	1
1/4 cup	chopped dried licorice root	50 mL
1 tbsp	ground dried ginseng root	15 mL

1. Scrub dandelion, burdock and chicory roots; finely chop in a food processor. Spread mixture on baking sheet; roast in preheated oven for 45 minutes, stirring after 20 minutes, until golden. Reduce oven temperature to 200° F (100° C); bake for 1 hour or until thoroughly dry, stirring every 20 minutes. Allow to cool.

2. Meanwhile, crush cinnamon stick using a mortar and pestle, food processor or blender.

3. In a bowl, combine roasted roots with cinnamon, licorice and ginseng. Transfer to an airtight jar to store. Roots must be thoroughly dried before storing.

TO BREW ROOT COFFEE:

Just before using, grind small amounts at a time with a mortar and pestle, coffee grinder or mini food processor. Use 1 tbsp (15 mL) ground roots for every 1 cup (250 mL) of water. Brew in a coffee maker as you would regular coffee.

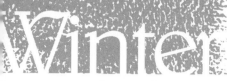

Hot Cinnamon Wine

Serves 4

Cinnamon is an antiseptic and has been used in Auyrvedic medicine as an expectorant and decongestant for the respiratory system.

Ginger is warming, while turmeric is antibacterial. When taken together as a winter drink, this beverage is an excellent way of diverting or treating a cold.

VARIATIONS

Omit: Turmeric root, if unavailable.

3 cups	red wine	750 mL
2	4-inch (10 cm) cinnamon sticks	2
1	1-inch (2.5 cm) piece ginger root, sliced	1
1	1-inch (2.5 cm) piece fresh turmeric root, sliced	1

1. In a non-reactive saucepan, add wine, cinnamon, ginger and turmeric. Cover and heat gently over medium heat. Remove from heat and allow to stand, covered, for 20 minutes.

2. Strain and pour into 4 heated mugs or glasses.

Condiments, Sauces & Dressings

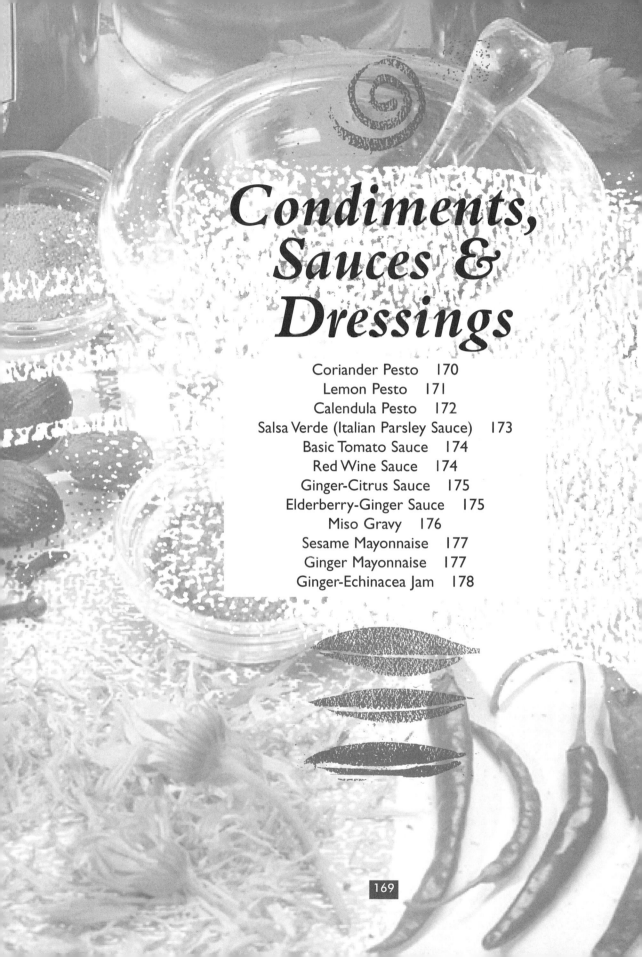

Coriander Pesto

**Makes 1 1/4 cups
(300 mL)**

VARIATIONS

Substitute: Flat-leafed
Italian parsley for
cilantro.

Healing Condiments
Prepared sauces, dips, spreads
and other convenience foods are
filled with additives, preservatives
and other refined foods. They
may be very harmful if taken
regularly and are usually the first
foods to be purged from the
refrigerator and shelves of people
wishing to move towards a
healthy diet. At the same time,
homemade condiments made
from chili, tomatoes, fruit and
other organic, garden-fresh veg-
etables and healing herbs can
add a concentrated dose of medic-
inal goodness to everyday meals.

2	cloves garlic	2
1 tbsp	finely crushed coriander seeds	15 mL
1	green chili pepper, quartered	1
1	bunch fresh cilantro, stems and leaves of upper half only	1
1/4 cup	pine nuts	50 mL
1/4 cup	freshly grated Parmesan cheese	50 mL
1/3 cup	olive oil	75 mL

1. In a food processor or blender, mince garlic with coriander seeds. Add chili pepper, cilantro, nuts and cheese. Process until minced. With motor running, add olive oil in a steady stream until well blended. Season to taste with salt and pepper if desired.

Lemon Pesto

Makes 1 cup (250 mL)

TIP

Some herbs have a natural lemon flavor — lemon balm, lemon grass, lemon verbena. Others have a specific lemon variety — basil, mint, sage, thyme. Use any of them in this recipe. Try this pesto in vegetable stir-fries, tossed with pasta, as a stuffing for fish or whisk 2 tbsp (25 mL) pesto with 1/2 cup (125 mL) olive oil and 3 tbsp (45 mL) rice or white vinegar for a light spring salad dressing.

VARIATIONS

Substitute: Thyme, savory, hyssop or tarragon for lemon herb.

3	large cloves garlic	3
1/4 cup	unblanched almonds	50 mL
2 cups	fresh basil leaves, firmly packed	500 mL
3 tbsp	chopped fresh lemon herb leaves (see Tip, at left)	45 mL
1/4 cup	freshly grated Parmesan cheese	50 mL
1 tsp	finely grated lemon zest	5 mL
1/4 cup	olive oil	50 mL
2 tbsp	lemon juice	25 mL

1. Mince garlic in a food processor or blender. Add almonds and process until coarsely chopped. Add basil, lemon herb, cheese and lemon zest; process until minced. With machine running, add oil and lemon juice in a steady stream. Process or blend until well mixed. Season to taste with salt and pepper if desired.

2. Transfer mixture to a jar or storage container. Cover and refrigerate for up to 2 days or feeeze for up to 1 month.

Calendula Pesto

**Makes 1 1/2 cups
(375 mL)**

TIP

Many summer flowers lend themselves to pestos. In this recipe, try the flower petals of echinacea, thyme, sage, rosemary, mint, hyssop and savory for a colorful pesto.

VARIATIONS

Substitute: 1/2-inch (1 cm) piece fresh ginger root for ginger in syrup; Any edible flower petals (see suggestions, above) for calendula.

2	garlic cloves	2
2	ginger squares in syrup	2
1/2 cup	unblanched almonds	125 mL
1 cup	fresh calendula petals	250 mL
1/2 cup	fresh basil leaves	125 mL
1/2 cup	fresh thyme leaves	125 mL
3/4 cup	freshly grated Parmesan cheese	175 mL
3/4 cup	olive oil	175 mL

1. In a food processor or blender, mince garlic and ginger for 1 minute. Add nuts; process until coarsely chopped. Add calendula, basil, thyme and cheese; process until minced. With motor running, add olive oil in a steady stream. Process or blend until well mixed. Season to taste with salt and pepper if desired.

2. Transfer mixture to a jar or storage container. Cover and refrigerate for up to 2 days or feeeze for up to 1 month.

Salsa Verde
(Italian Parsley Sauce)

**Makes 1 1/2 to 2 cups
(375 to 500 mL)**

TIP

Serve this versatile, healthy sauce as a spread for crackers or bread, a dip for fresh vegetables, or as a sauce over cooked lentils, steamed vegetables, chicken or fish.

VARIATIONS

Substitute: Hyssop leaves for alfalfa; Sage for rosemary; 3 tbsp (45 mL) dried alfalfa for fresh; Any herbed vinegar for healing vinegar.

2	day-old, whole grain bread slices, crusts removed, torn into pieces	2
3 tbsp	healing vinegar	45 mL
1/4 cup	chopped fresh rosemary	50 mL
3	cloves garlic	3
3 cups	packed fresh parsley leaves	750 mL
1/2 cup	chopped fresh alfalfa	125 mL
6	anchovies, chopped	6
3/4 to 1 cup	extra-virgin olive oil	175 to 250 mL

1. In a small bowl, toss bread with vinegar. Allow to sit for a few minutes to soften bread.

2. In a food processor or blender, process rosemary and garlic until minced. Add parsley, alfalfa and anchovies. Process until finely chopped. Add bread; process to blend. With motor running, add oil in a steady stream until sauce reaches desired consistency — thicker for spreads, slightly thinner for dips and thinner still for sauces. Season to taste with salt and pepper if desired. May be made 1 day ahead and kept covered in the refrigerator.

Basic Tomato Sauce

Makes 8 cups (2 L)

TIP

Tomatoes are ripe and ready in the fall for fresh salads. But making this sauce saves the harvest for use all winter. For best consistency, use plum or paste tomatoes. You can freeze the sauce in 2-cup (500 mL) containers.

4 tbsp	olive oil	50 mL
5	cloves garlic, minced	5
3	onions, chopped	3
30	plum tomatoes (or 15 large field tomatoes), cut into eighths	30
6	sprigs fresh oregano	6
6	sprigs fresh thyme	6
6	sprigs fresh basil	6

1. In a large pot, heat oil over medium heat. Add garlic and onion; sauté for 5 minutes or until soft. Add tomatoes, oregano, thyme and basil; cover and bring to a boil. Reduce heat and simmer for 2 hours, uncovering after tomatoes have released juices. Cook, stirring occasionally until thick and reduced to about half. Season to taste with salt and pepper if desired.

2. Allow sauce to cool. Strain liquid off, pressing vegetables to release goodness.

Red Wine Sauce

Makes about 1 cup (250 mL)

TIP

Serve with vegetables, grains or or vegetable patties.

VARIATIONS

Substitute: Other fruit or herbal syrups for elderberry syrup.

1 tbsp	olive oil	15 mL
1 tbsp	butter	15 mL
1 cup	finely chopped onions	250 mL
1 1/4 cups	red wine	300 mL
1 tbsp	chopped fresh thyme leaves	15 mL
1 tbsp	elderberry syrup	15 mL

1. In a medium saucepan, heat oil and butter over medium heat. Add onions and cook, stirring occasionally, for 8 minutes or until soft.

2. Add wine. Adjust heat to keep sauce simmering and cook for 15 minutes or until reduced to 1 cup (250 mL).

3. Stir in thyme and syrup; cook for another 2 minutes. Serve warm or at room temperature. Keep in refrigerator to serve as a condiment.

Ginger-Citrus Sauce

**Makes 3/4 cup
(175 mL)**

TIP

Use this as a dipping sauce or toss with a salad.

VARIATIONS

Substitute: Lemon juice for orange juice; Healing or herbed vinegar for rice vinegar; Thyme leaves and 1 tsp (5 mL) lemon zest for lemon thyme.

3 tbsp	chopped ginger root	45 mL
1	small jalapeno pepper, seeded and quartered	1
1/4 cup	lemon thyme leaves	50 mL
3 tbsp	fresh sage leaves	45 mL
1/3 cup	fresh orange juice	75 mL
1 tbsp	soya sauce	15 mL
1 tbsp	rice vinegar	15 mL
2 tbsp	smooth peanut butter	25 mL
1 tbsp	sesame oil	25 mL

1. In a food processor or blender, mince ginger and jalapeno pepper. Add thyme and sage; process to mince. With motor running, add juice, soya sauce, vinegar, peanut butter and sesame oil. Process until mixture is smooth. Season to taste with salt and pepper if desired. Serve at room temperature.

Elderberry-Ginger Sauce

Makes 3 cups (750 mL)

TIP

A healing sauce for winter. Great with stir-fries and vegetable rice dishes.

VARIATIONS

Substitute: Any herb jelly for elderberry jelly; Chopped preserved ginger for burdock in syrup; If fresh ginseng root is not available, simmer 1 dried ginseng root in water for 15 minutes, then mince. (Reserve cooking water for tea).

2 tbsp	olive oil	25 mL
1 tbsp	minced ginger root	15 mL
1 tbsp	minced fresh ginseng root	15 mL
2 tbsp	whole wheat flour	25 mL
1 cup	stock	250 mL
2 tbsp	soya sauce	25 mL
2 tbsp	cider vinegar	25 mL
3 tbsp	finely chopped burdock root in syrup	45 mL
1/2 cup	elderberry jelly	125 mL
1 cup	MISO GRAVY (see recipe, page 176)	250 mL

1. In a saucepan, heat oil over medium–low heat. Add ginger and ginseng and cook, stirring often, for 3 minutes. Stir in flour; cook stirring, for 2 minutes.
2. Add stock, soya sauce, vinegar, burdock, elderberry jelly and gravy. Increase heat to simmer gently for 10 minutes. Serve warm. Keeps in refrigerator for up to 3 days.

Miso Gravy

TIP

Miso is a thick, salty paste made from cooked, aged soybeans and often grains. It is used as a flavoring and for soup bases and is available in darker or lighter varieties.

VARIATIONS

Substitute: 2 tbsp (25 mL) red wine vinegar for red wine (increase stock to 2 cups [500 mL]); Tomato paste for miso.

1 tbsp	olive oil	15 mL
1 tsp	cumin seeds	5 mL
2	cloves garlic, finely chopped	2
1/2 cup	finely chopped onions	125 mL
1/2 cup	chopped shiitake mushrooms	125 mL
2 tbsp	chopped fresh thyme leaves	25 mL
2 tbsp	chopped fresh sage leaves	25 mL
2 tbsp	chopped fresh parsley	25 mL
1 tbsp	sesame oil	15 mL
1/4 cup	whole wheat flour	50 mL
1 1/2 cups	stock	375 mL
1/2 cup	red wine	125 mL
3 tbsp	red or brown miso	45 mL

1. In a medium saucepan, heat olive oil over medium-low heat. Add cumin seeds, and cook, stirring, for 1 minute. Add garlic and onions; cook, stirring occasionally, for 5 minutes. Stir in mushrooms, thyme, sage and parsley. Cook for 10 minutes or until mixture is soft.

2. Stir in sesame oil and flour. Remove pan from heat. Stir in stock and wine. Set heat to simmer and cook for 5 minutes or until mixture thickens. Stir in miso. Remove from heat and serve.

Sesame Mayonnaise

**Makes about 1 cup
(250 mL)**

TIP

Sesame oil adds a roast-
ed, smoky taste to dips
and sauces. Use in small
quantities.

VARIATIONS

Substitute: White vinegar
for rice vinegar.

1	egg	1
1 tbsp	rice vinegar	15 mL
1 tbsp	Dijon mustard	15 mL
1 tbsp	soya sauce	15 mL
3/4 cup	olive oil	150 mL
2 tbsp	toasted sesame oil	25 mL

1. In a food processor or blender, add egg, vinegar, mustard and soya sauce. Process until combined.

2. With motor running, slowly add olive oil and sesame oil in a steady stream until blended and thick. Mixture will thicken when chilled.

Ginger Mayonnaise

Makes 1 cup (250 mL)

TIP

This is a lower-fat
alternative to regular
mayonnaise. Set natural
yogurt over a strainer
lined with cheesecloth;
drain into a bowl for at
least 3 hours in refrigerator. Use homemade
mayonnaise for best
results.

VARIATIONS

Substitute: White wine
for healing white wine.

1/2 cup	mayonnaise	125 mL
1/2 cup	drained yogurt (see Tip, at left)	125 mL
1 tbsp	healing white wine (see pages 44–45)	15 mL
1 tsp	ground ginger	5 mL
1/2 tsp	turmeric	2 mL
1/4 cup	minced crystallized or preserved ginger	50 mL

1. In a small bowl, whisk together mayonnaise and yogurt until smooth. Whisk in wine, ginger and turmeric. Stir in ginger; cover and refrigerate for at least 1 hour to blend flavors.

Ginger-Echinacea Jam

Makes 3 cups (750 mL)

In 1980, a Cornell Medical School researcher observed that his blood didn't clot and traced the cause to his regular consumption of a marmalade that contained 15% ginger. This led him to study ginger's ability to inhibit platelet clumping.

TIP

To test if jam is set, drop 1/2 tsp (2 mL) on a chilled plate. Place in the freezer for 2 minutes. Remove and tilt the plate; if the jam holds its shape, it is set. If not, continue to cook.

Roots should be fresh for this recipe; if echinacea is not available, try fresh burdock or dandelion root in its place.

VARIATIONS

Substitute: Brown rice syrup for honey.

2 cups	chopped peeled ginger root	500 mL
1 cup	chopped fresh echinacea root	250 mL
2 cups	water	500 mL
3/4 cup	honey	150 mL
1 cup	granulated sugar	250 mL
1/4 cup	chopped thyme leaves	50 mL

1. In a blender, process chopped roots and water until fine.

2. Transfer to a large saucepan. Stir in honey and sugar; boil over medium-high heat, stirring occasionally, for 10 to 15 minutes or until softly set.

3. Stir in thyme; cook 1 minute. Pour into a clean jar; cover when cool. Store in refrigerator.

ORGANIZATIONS

Canadian Herb Society
5251 Oak Street, Vancouver, BC, V6M
4H1 Canada
Tel (604) 222 3488
Fax (604) 222 9613
allison@imag.net, www.herbsociety.ca

Herb Society of America, Inc.
9019 Kirtland Chardon Road, Kirtland,
Ohio 44094, USA
Tel (440)2560514
Fax (440) 256 0541
herbsociet@aol.com
www.herbsociety.org

International Herb Association
PO Box 317, Mundelein, IL 60060, USA
Tel (847) 949 4372
Fax (847) 949 5896

HERBS AND SEEDS

Garden Escape
Tel 1 800 466 8142,
Fax (512) 472 6645
www.garden.com
*Internet-based gardening resource; over
10,000 gardening products and sources for
herb plants and seeds.*

Gilbertie's Herb Gardens
7 Sylvan Lane, Westport, Connecticut,
USA
Largest herb plant supplier in the USA.

Logee's Greenhouses
141 North Street, Danielson, Ct 06239,
USA
Tel (860) 774 8038
Fax (860) 774 9932
www.logees.com
Rare plants, herbs and seeds; catalog $3.

Redwood City Seed Company
P.O. Box 361, Redwood City, CA 94064,
USA
Tel (650) 325 7333
www.batnet.com/rwc-seed
*Southwestern and Mexican seeds and plants;
catalog.*

Richters
Goodwood, Ontario, L0C 1A0, Canada
Tel (905) 640 6677
Fax (905) 640 6641
www.richters.com
*Herb specialists, mail order: seeds, plants,
books; catalog..*

Sandy Mush Herb Nursery
316 Surrett Cove Rd., Leicester, N.C.
28748-5517, USA
Tel (828) 683 2014
Plants and seeds; catalog $4.

Southern Perennials and Herbs
98 Bridges Road, Tylertown, MS 39667 -
9338, USA
Tel 1 (800) 774 0079
Tel (601) 684 1769
Fax (601) 684 3729
www.s-p-h.com
Plants and seeds; catalog.

The Cooks Garden
P.O. Box 5010, Hodges, SC 29653, USA
Tel 1 800 457 9703
www.cooksgarden.com
*Seeds and supplies for kitchen gardeners;
catalog.*

Well-Sweep Herb Farm
205 Mt Bethel Road, Port Murray, NJ
07865 USA
Tel (908) 852 5390
Plants and seeds; catalog $2.

A Modern Herbal
Mrs. M. Grieve, Mrs. C.F. Leyel, editor,
New York, U.S.A.: Dover Publications
Inc., 1971; two volumes, unabridged
republication of original (1931) edition.
ISBN: 0-486-22798-7

Healing with Herbal Juices
Siegfried Gursche, Vancouver, B.C.,
Canada: Alive Books, 1993.
ISBN: 0-920470-34-3

Herbal Tonics
Daniel B. Mowrey, Ph.D., New Canaan,
Connecticut, U.S.A.: Keats Publishing,
Inc., 1993.
ISBN: 0-87983-565-6

Meals That Heal
Lisa Turner, Rochester, Vermont, U.S.A.:
Healing Arts Press, 1996.
ISBN: 0-89281-625-2

Medicinal Mushrooms
Christopher Hobbs, Capitola, CA,
U.S.A.: Botanica Press, 1996.
ISBN: 1-884-36001-7

**Rodale's Basic Natural Foods
Cookbook**
Charles Gerras, Ed., Emmaus, PA, U.S.A.:
Rodale Press, 1984.
ISBN: 0-87857-469-7

The Complete Medicinal Herbal
Penelope Ody, Great Britain: Dorling
Kindersley Limited, 1993.
ISBN: 1-55013-480-9

The Grains Cookbook
Bert Greene, New York, NY, U.S.A.:
Workman Publishing, 1988.
ISBN: 0-89480-610-6

The Green Pharmacy
James A. Duke, PhD, Emmaus, PA,
U.S.A.: Rodale Press, 1997.
ISBN: 0-312-96648-2

The New Holistic Herbal
David Hoffman, Rockport MA, U.S.A.:
Element Inc., 1992.
ISBN: 1-85230-193-7

The Sea Vegetable Book
Judith Cooper Madlener, New York, NY,
U.S.A.: Clarkson N. Potter, Inc. 1977.
ISBN: 0-517-52906-8

Adaptogen. A substance that builds resistance to stress by balancing the functions of the glands and immune system, thus strengthening the immune system, nervous system, and glandular system. Adaptogens promote overall vitality. *Some adaptogen herbs:* astragalus, ginseng.

Analgesic. A substance that receives pain by acting as a nervine, antiseptic or counterirritant. *Some analgesic herbs:* echinacea, turmeric.

Anodyne. Herbs that relieve pain. *Some anodyne herbs:* clove.

Antibiotic. Meaning "against life," antibiotics are substances that work to terminate the life of infectious agents, including bacteria and fungi, without endangering the patient's health. Modern antibiotics are powerless against viral infections and may actually suppress our natural resistance to viruses. *Some antibiotic herbs:* garlic, green tea, lavender, sage, thyme.

Anti-Inflammatory. Controlling or reducing swelling, redness, pain and heat which is a reaction of the body to injury or infection. *Some anti-inflammatory herbs:* chamomile, St. John's wort.

Antimicrobial. Herbs that kill or suppresses the growth of bacteria and other microorganisms. *Some antimicrobial herbs:* turmeric, thyme, peppermint, rosemary, sage, cayenne, cinnamon, cloves, echinacea, coriander, garlic, lavender, licorice, calendula, St. John's wort.

Antioxidant. A compound that protects cells by preventing polyunsaturated fatty acids (PUFFAs) in cell membranes from oxidizing, or breaking down. They do this by neutralizing free radicals. *Some antioxidant herbs:* alfalfa, dandelion leaves, ginseng, parsley, garlic, watercress. *Some antioxidant foods:* fresh asparagus, beet tops, walnuts.

Antineoplastic. Herbs that inhibit and combat the development of tumors.

Antiseptic. Herbs used to prevent or counteract the growth of disease germs. *Some antiseptic herbs:* rosemary, thyme.

Antispasmodic. Herbal remedies that rapidly relax nervous tension which may be causing digestive spasms of colic. *Some antispasmodic herbs:* lavender, rosemary, thyme, chamomile, ginger.

Astringent. Substances that aid in breaking down secretions. *Some astringent herbs:* calendula, cinnamon, thyme

BHA. A chemical added to foods to help preserve them; may possibly cause elevated cholesterol, liver and kidney damage.

Cathartic. Herbs that have a laxative effort.

Carminative. Herbs that sooth the digestive tract and are taken to relieve gas and gripe. *Some carminative herbs:* allspice, cloves, caraway, dill, fennel, horsebalm, peppermint, sage, thyme.

Catarrh gargle. To make a strong tea of the herb, when cool use as a gargle. *Some gargle herbs:* sage, thyme

Cholagogue. Promotes the flow and discharge of bile into the small intestine.

Cruciferous. Cabbage (including bok choy), cauliflower, some greens (collard, kale, mustard), rutabagas and turnips are all plants with cross-shaped flower petals, or cruciferous. Shown by research to be extremely active in preventing cancer, cruciferous vegetables should be eaten at least 4 times per week.

Decoction. A solution obtained by using the woody parts of plants (roots, seeds, bark) and boiling them in water ten to 20 minutes.

Demulcent. Soothing substances taken internally to protect damaged tissue. *Some demulcent herbs:* marsh mallow, fenugreek.

Designer foods. Processed foods that are supplemented with food ingredients high in disease-preventing substances. These foods do not take the place of natural foods.

Diaphoretic. Herbs used to induce sweating. *Some diaphoretic herbs:* cayenne, chamomile, cinnamon, ginger

Diuretic. Herbs that increase the flow of urine, meant to be used for short term only. *Some diuretic herbs:* dandelion leaf and root, burdock, linden, pumpkin seed.

Dysmenorrhea. Condition of menstruation accompanied by cramping pains which may be incapacitating in their intensity.

Elixir. A tonic that invigorates or strengthens the body by stimulating or restoring health.

Emmenagogue. Herbs that promote menstruation.

Some herbs that act as an emmenagogue: calendula, chamomile.

Essential oil. The oil derived by distillation from flowers, leaves, stems of plants.

Expectorant. Herbs that help to relieve congestion from colds. *Some expectorant herbs:* elder, garlic, ginger, hyssop.

Fortified foods. Foods with added nutrients to restore those lost in processing or to prevent nutritional deficiencies.

Free radicals. Unstable compounds that scavenge oxygen from healthy cells, often destroying them. Most major chronic disease and the aging process are linked to free radical damage. Free radicals are a result of external agents such a radiation, cigarette smoke, exhaust fumes, injury, disease and poor nutrition.

Hepatic. Herbs that strengthen, tone and stimulate secretive functions of the liver. *Some hepatic herbs:* turmeric.

Laxative. Herbs that stimulate bowel movement, meant to be used for short term only.

Miso. A thick, salty paste made from cooked, aged soy-

beans and often grains; used for flavoring and soup bases.

Mutagenesis. The process whereby cells are mutated or changed into cancerous cells.

Nervine. Herbs used to ease anxiety and stress and nourish the nerves. *Some nervine herbs:* chamomile, valerian, thyme.

Non-reactive cooking utensils. The acids in foods can react with certain materials and promote the oxidation of some nutrients and discoloration. Non-reactive materials suitable for brewing teas and preparing jams and jellies are: glass, enamel-coated cast iron or stainless steel, and stainless steel. While cast iron pans are recommended for cooking (a meal cooked in unglazed cast iron can provide 20 percent of the total daily iron intake), it is not recommended for brewing teas.

Organosulfides. Compounds that have been shown to reduce blood pressure, lower cholesterol levels, and reduce blood clotting. *Some herbs/foods that contain organosulfides:* garlic, onions.

Phytochemicals. Chemicals from a plant. *Phyto*, from the Greek, means "to bring forth," and is used as a prefix to designate "from a plant."

Purgative. Substances that promote bowel movement and increased intestinal peristalsis.

Rhizome. Underground stem, usually thick and fleshy.

Rice syrup. A thick, sweet syrup made from rice, preferably brown rice.

Rubefacient. Herbs that, when applied to the skin, stimulate circulation in that area. *Some rubefacient herbs:* cayenne.

Scape. Long green stem growing from garlic bud; appears in early summer with flower bud. Flower bud and tender green stem are edible.

Sedative. Herbs that have a powerful quieting effect on the nervous system to relieve tension and induce sleep. *Some sedative herbs:* valerian, chamomile, linden, lavender

Styptic. Herbs causing capillaries to contract and thereby stop superficial hemorrhage bleeding.

Tahini. A thick, smooth paste made from raw, ground sesame seeds.

Tamari. A naturally brewed wheat-free soya sauce that contains no sugar.

Tempeh. A high-protein, cultured food made from soybeans, often only available frozen.

Therapeutic dose. Amounts recommended by herbalists for healing certain ailments, usually higher and for longer periods of time than herbs used in cooking for maintaining health.

Tincture. Liquid herbal extracts made by soaking an herb in a solvent (usually alcohol) to extract the plant's constituents. Some herbalists maintain that because tinctures contain a wide range of the plant's chemical constituents and they are one of the most easily absorbed forms of herbs, they are the best way to take herbs.

Tisane. The correct term used for steeping fresh or dried herbs in boiling water. Interchangeable with "tea" when herbs are used.

Tonic. Tonic herbs support the body's systems in maintaining health. Depending on what herbs are used, they can support the whole body or specific systems or organs. They are able to do this because they contain opposing groups of constituents that can lower or raise, stimulate or depress, increase or decrease individual biological processes. Tonics increase the tone of the body tissues, imparting strength and vitality by; promoting the digestive process, improving blood circulation, increasing the supply of oxygen to the tissues. Tonic herbs are safe to use daily. *Some tonic herbs:* alfalfa (nutritive tonic for musculoskeletal system), yarrow (digestive tonic), devil's claw (liver tonic), licorice root, echinacea (immune system tonic), dandelion (general tonic, liver and digestive tonic).

Vasodilator. An herb that relaxes blood vessels which benefits in increasing circulation by bringing blood to the peripheries (e.g. arms, hands, legs, feet, brain). *Some vasodilator herbs:* peppermint, sage.

Vermifuge. Herbs taken to kill worms in the intestine.

Vulnerary. An herbal remedy that brings about wound healing and reduces inflammation. *Some vulnerary herbs:* calendula.

Eggplant:
   fruit-stuffed, 133
   lasagna, 116-17
   manicotti with spinach pesto stuffing, 105
   vegetable paella, 106
Eggs:
   raw, about, 55
   vegetable frittata, 61
Eight-treasure noodle pot, 145
Elderberry, -ginger sauce, 175
Enchiladas, 110-11

F

Fall fruit en papillotte, 156
Fall vegetable paella, 106
Fennel, about, 108
Feta cheese, chive and dandelion dip, 51
Fettucine, and fiddleheads in thyme vinaigrette, 140
Fiddleheads, fettucine and, 140
Fish:
   cakes, 113
   noodle pot, 145
Flowers:
   edible, 85
   and pestos, 172
   summer salad, 85
Frittata, vegetable, 61
Fruit:
   en papillotte, 156
   gingered summer, 154
   -stuffed roasted eggplant, 133
   See also specific fruits

Fruited pesto-pasta, 57

G

Garlic:
   preserving, 59
   to roast, 88
   and rosemary stuffed mushrooms, 53
Gazpacho, calendula-strawberry, 72
Geranium, about lemon-scented, 121
Ginger:
   -citrus sauce, 175
   -echinacea jam, 178
   -elderberry sauce, 175
   mayonnaise, 177
   sun tea, 165
Ginger ale, ginseng, 164
Gingerbread, 157
Gingered summer fruit, 154
Ginseng:
   -ginger ale, 164
   meusli, 60
Goat cheese:
   with tomatoes and pesto, 131
   warm mushroom salad, 82
Golden lemon thyme, about, 121
Gravy, miso, 176
Green tea:
   sauce, 154
   and summer flower blend, 165
Green tomato and apple salsa, 110-11

Grilled portobello mushroom salad, 91

H

Healing condiments, 170
Herbed fresh pasta, 141
Hijiki, spinach and sea vegetable soup, 69
Hot-and-sour summer soup, 70
Hot mulled wine and elderberry, 166
Hot spiced apple cider, 166
Hot sweet potato salad, 94

I

Immune-spiced soba noodle salad, 143
Italian parsley sauce, 173

J

Jam, ginger-echinacea, 178
Jambalaya, 98
Julienne strips, to prepare, 89

K

Kamut:
   with sautéed summer vegetables, 142
   -vegetable pilaf, 144
Kohlrabi, tomato soup, 80

L

Lambsquarter, with almond butter sauce, 84
Lasagna, winter vegetable, 116-17

Lavosh, about, 97

Lavender aïoli, 54-55

Leeks:

    about, 130

    and mushroom pilaf, 137

    onion and garlic tart, 50

    vegetable pot pie, 114-15

Lemon balm, about, 121

Lemongrass, about, 121

Lemon herbs, about, 121

Lemon pesto, 171

Lentils, and cracked wheat wrap, 118

Lima beans:

    corn and rice chowder, 73

    and cracked wheat wrap, 118

Linguine, with caramelized onions and leeks, 136

M

Maitake mushroom cream soup, 66

Mayonnaise:

    and aïoli, 55

    ginger, 177

    sesame, 177

Mesclun:

    about, 82

    warm mushroom salad, 82

Meusli, 60

Miso:

    about, 71

    gravy, 176

Moroccan squash, 129

Mountain bread, about, 97

Mousse, strawberry, 151

Mushrooms:

    -almond bisque, 71

    cream soup, 66

    stuffed with garlic and rosemary, 53

Mustard greens, wild rice baked with, 138

N

Noodle pot, eight-treasure, 146

O

Okra, gumbo, 76

Onions:

    about, 79

    See also Caramelized onions

P

Parchment paper, about, 156

Parsley persillade, 73

Parsnips:

    calendula-glazed, 134

    vegetable cakes, 113

    vegetable ragout, 107

Pasta:

    broccoli-pesto salad, 86

    with caramelized onions and leeks, 136

    and fiddleheads in thyme vinaigrette, 140

    fruit pesto, 57

    herbed fresh, 141

Pâté, vegetable, 56

Peaches, rose compote, 152

Pears:

    with apricot ginger sauce, 155

    spiced salsa, 160

Pesto:

    calendula, 172

    coriander, 170

    lemon, 171

    roasted garlic and red pepper, 59

    spinach, 105

    stuffed squash flowers, 124

Pilaf:

    kamut-vegetable, 144

    leek and mushroom, 137

Pita, about, 97

Poached cherries with rosemary custard, 153

Poached pears with apricot ginger sauce, 155

Portobello mushrooms:

    kamut-vegetable pilaf, 144

    salad, 91

    stuffed with garlic and rosemary, 53

Potato(es):

    about, 86

    baked with onions and leek, 130

    braised with cabbage, 108-9

    braised with spring vegetables, 120

    and celeriac au gratin, 128

    leek and onion tart, 50

    and red lentil salad, 87

    salad, 94

Potato(es) (continued):

    scalloped with turnips, 122

    vegetable pot pie, 114–15

Q

Quinoa, with couscous and cranberries, 145

R

Red lentil and potato salad, 87

Red wine sauce, 174

Refried beans, enchiladas, 110–11

Rhubarb:

    about, 141

    -strawberry crêpes, 150

Rice:

    leek and mushroom pilaf, 137

    stuffed squash flowers, 124

    tomatoes stuffed with mushrooms and, 126

    vegetable sushi, 62–63

    See also Brown rice; Wild rice

Roasted garlic:

    and black bean spread, 52

    and red pepper pesto, 59

Roasted red peppers:

    in marinade, 58

    with wild rice and walnuts, 127

Roasted squash:

    onion and garlic soup, 78

    and pepper salad, 88

Roasted vegetable and tomato bouillabaisse, 75

Root coffee, 167

Root vegetables, and Cheddar soup, 77

Rosemary:

    custard, 153

    and garlic stuffed mushrooms, 53

Rutabaga:

    vegetable cakes, 113

    vegetable pot pie, 114–15

Rutubaga, tomato soup, 80

S

Salad:

    autumn harvest, 89

    beet and feta cheese, 93

    broccoli-pesto, 86

    dandelion, 83

    grilled portobello mushroom, 91

    hot sweet potato, 94

    lambsquarter, 84

    potato and red lentil, 87

    roasted squash and pepper, 88

    soba noodle, 143

    summer flower, 85

    sweet-and-sour beet, 90

    wakame-cabbage, 92

    of warm wild mushrooms, 82

Salad greens:

    with almond butter sauce, 84

    and flower salad, 85

Salsa:

    green tomato and apple, 110–11

    spiced pear, 160

    verde, 173

Sauces:

    almond butter, 84

    apricot ginger, 155

    barbecue, 102–3

    ginger-citrus, 175

    green tea, 154

    Italian parsley, 173

    red wine, 174

    sesame, 148

    spring, 123

    tomato, 174

Scalloped turnips with potatoes and onion, 122

Scallops:

    gumbo, 76

    noodle pot, 145

Scapes, cauliflower with split peas, 125

Sea gumbo, 76

Sea vegetables, and spinach soup, 69

Sesame:

    mayonnaise, 177

    sauce, 148

Sesame seeds, about, 148

Sheep sorrel:

    about, 123

    spring sauce, 123

Shiitake mushrooms:

    cream soup, 66

    lasagna, 116–17

    and leek pilaf, 137

Shiitake mushrooms (cont.):

roasted peppers stuffed with wild rice and, 127

stir-fried with vegetables, 99

summer soup, 70

tomatoes stuffed with, 126

warm salad of, 82

Shrimp:

gumbo, 76

noodle pot, 145

Smoothies, strawberry banana, 162

Snow peas, braised spring vegetables, 120

Soba noodles, about, 143

Sorrel, wild rice baked with, 138

Soup:

Cheddar cheese and root vegetables, 77

cold, calendula-strawberry gazpacho, 72

corn and rice chowder, 73

curried yam, 74

hot-and-sour summer, 70

mushroom, cream of, 66

mushroom-almond bisque, 71

roasted squash, onion and garlic, 78

sea gumbo, 76

spinach and sea vegetable, 69

tomato-thyme, 80

vegetable and tomato bouillabaisse, 75

Spelt:

chickpea-herb burgers, 104

corn-zucchini beet casseroles, 100

Spiced pear salsa, 160

Spice paste, 132

Spinach:

dandelion salad with citrus dressing, 83

feta and chive dip, 51

pesto, 105

and sea vegetable soup, 69

spring sauce, 123

vegetable frittata, 61

warm sweet-and-sour beet salad, 90

Split peas, with cauliflower, 125

Spring sauce, 123

Spring tonic, 163

about, 163

broth, 68

Spring vegetables, with citrus dressing, 120

Squash:

baked Moroccan, 129

leek and onion tart, 50

Squash flowers, stuffed, 124

Starters:

black bean and roasted garlic spread, 52

feta, chive and dandelion dip, 51

fruited pesto-pasta, 57

garlic and rosemary stuffed mushrooms, 53

ginseng meusli, 60

Starters (continued):

leek, onion and garlic tart, 50

roasted garlic and red pepper pesto, 59

roasted red peppers in marinade, 58

sweet potato crisps with lavender aïoli, 54

vegetable frittata, 61

See also Pâté

Stir fry, vegetables with bulgur, 99

Strawberry:

banana smoothie, 162

-calendula gazpacho, 72

mousse, 151

Stuffed braised cabbage with potatoes, 108-9

Summer flower salad, 85

Sushi, vegetable, 62-63

Sweet potato(es):

crisps with lavender aïoli, 54

leek and onion tart, 50

salad, 94

scalloped with turnips, 122

vegetable pot pie, 114-15

vegetable sushi, 62-63

Swiss chard, spring sauce, 123

T

Tahini, to make, 148

Tarts, leek, onion and garlic, 50

Lovage, about, 67

M

Maitake mushroom, about, 26–27

Marsh marigold, about, 67

Matricaria recutita, 14–15

Medicago sativa, 11

Medicinal herbs, cooking with, 35–47

Memory-boosting seasoning, 44

Mentha piperita, 28–29

Mushrooms, about, 26–27

N

Nori, about, 31

Nuts and seeds, about, 47

O

Oils, about, 41–42

P

Palmaria palmata, 31

Panax ginseng, 22–23

   P. quinquefolius, 22–23

Parsley, about, 27–28

Peppermint, about, 28–29

Petroselinum crispum, 27–28

Pleurophycus gardneri, 31

Porphyra tenera, 31

Pot herb, about, 67

R

Raspberry, about, 34

Red clover, about, 34

Roots, crystallized, 40

Rose, about, 34

Rosemary, about, 29–30

Rosmarinus officinalis, 29–30

Rubus idaeus, 34

S

Sage, about, 30

St. John's Wort, about, 34

Salvia officinalis, 30

Sambucus nigra, 18–19

Sea herbs, 31

Seasonings, herbal, 43

Seeds and nuts, about, 47

Shiitake mushrooms, about, 26–27

Soups, healing, 42–43

Soybeans, about, 46

Soy foods, 46–47

Sprouts, about, 47

Stevia, about, 34

Stinging nettle, about, 67

Syrups, about, 39

T

Taraxacum officinale, 16–17

Teas:

   digestive, 37

   healing herbal, 38

   medicinal, 36–38

   pain-reducing, 37

   stress-reducing, 37

Tempeh, about, 46–47

Thyme, about, 32

Tilia x *europaea*, 37

Tinctures, about, 38–39

Tofu, about, 46

Trifolium pratense, 34

Turmeric, about, 32–33

U

Undaria pinnatifida, 31

Urtica dioica, 67

V

Vinegars, healing, 40–41

W

Wakame, about, 31

Wild leeks, about, 67

Wines, 44–45

Z

Zingiber officinale, 21–22